Voice Science
Acoustics and Recording

Voice Science
Acoustics and Recording

David M. Howard, Ph.D.
Damian T. Murphy, Ph.D.

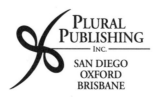

PLURAL
PUBLISHING
INC.
SAN DIEGO
OXFORD
BRISBANE

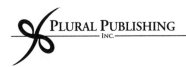

PLURAL PUBLISHING
INC.

5521 Ruffin Road
San Diego, CA 92123

e-mail: info@pluralpublishing.com
Web site: http://www.pluralpublishing.com

49 Bath Street
Abingdon, Oxfordshire OX14 1EA
United Kingdom

Typeset in 10½/13 Palatino Book by Flanagan's Publishing Services, Inc.
Printed in the United States of America by Bang Printing

For permission to use material from this text, contact us by
Telephone: (866) 758-7251
Fax: (888) 758-7255
e-mail: permissions@pluralpublishing.com

*Every attempt has been made to contact the copyright holders for material originally printed
in another source. If any have been inadvertently overlooked, the publishers will gladly make
the necessary arrangements at the first opportunity.*

Library of Congress Cataloging-in-Publication Data:

Howard, David M. (David Martin), 1956-
  Voice science, acoustics and recording / David M. Howard and Damien Murphy.
     p. cm.
  ISBN-13: 978-1-59756-078-8 (pbk.)
  ISBN-10: 1-59756-078-2 (pbk.)
 1. Voice. 2. Sound. 3. Sound--Recording and reproducing. I. Murphy, Damien
(Damien T.) II. Title.
  QP306.H77 2007
  612.7'8--dc22
                                                              2007036493

Contents

Preface   ix

1. INTRODUCTION   **1**
Overall Scope   1
Introductory Acoustics   2
    Numbers Large and Small   3
    Sound Transmission and Velocity   5
    Waveforms   8
    Sine Waves and Harmonics   10
    Short-Term and Long-Term Average Spectra   12
    Spectrograms   15
    Decibels   18
The Performer's Voice   21
Summary   21
Further Reading   23

2. THE HUMAN VOICE   **25**
Introduction   25
Voice Production   26
    Power Source in Voice Production   26
    Sound Source in Voice Production   29
    Sound Modifiers in Voice Production   33
    Voice   34
    Place   36
    Manner   38
Acoustics of the Vocal Output   38
    Power Source and Sound Source   38
    The Sound Modifiers   45
    Perturbation Theory   51
    Formants in Singing   53
Developing and Maintaining a Healthy Professional Voice   56
    Computers in Voice Training   56
    Tips for Maintaining a Healthy Voice   60
    Maintaining a Healthy Voice—Summary   63
Summary   64
Further Reading   64

3. THE VOICE ON LOCATION 67
Introduction 67
Acoustics of Spaces 68
  Introduction 68
  Sound Source into a Space 69
  Sound Modification by a Space 72
  Sound Output from a Space 75
Modifying the Acoustics of a Space 78
  Introduction 78
  Acoustics of Surface Materials 78
  Calculating Reverberation Time for a Room 80
  Changing Surface Materials in a Space 84
Performing to Best Acoustic Advantage in a Space 85
  Introduction 85
  Acoustic, Visual, and Practical Considerations 86
  Working the Space to Best Acoustic Advantage 86
  Vocal Performance Considerations 88
Summary 91
Further Reading 91

4. AUDIO SYSTEM FUNDAMENTALS 93
Introduction 93
Microphones 94
  Introduction 94
  Microphone Directivity Patterns 98
  Microphone Frequency Response 102
  Other Important Microphone Considerations 105
  Microphone Summary 107
Voice Recording Systems 108
  Introduction 108
  The Microphone Preamp Stage 108
  Conditioning the Signal Further—Inserts and EQ 113
  Interfacing with External Devices—The Auxiliary Section 117
  Routing and Output 119
  Hearing the Result—The Group Outputs and Master Section 120
  Insert Effects 122
  Aux Send Effects 127
  The Recording Medium 130
Vocal Sound Reinforcement 133
  Introduction 133
  Small Venues 134
  Medium Sized Venues 137
  Large Venues/More Complex Sound Reinforcement Systems 138
  Operational Guidelines 138
Summary 145
Further Reading 145

5. PRACTICAL VOICE RECORDING AND REINFORCEMENT   147

Introduction   147
Single Vocal Sources   149
  Introduction   149
  Recording for Research   149
  Studio Vocal Recording   150
  Live Vocal Sound Reinforcement   155
  Spoken Word   158
  Recording on Location   160
  Anechoic Recording   162
Multiple Vocal Sources   164
  Introduction   164
  Stereo Recording   164
  Multiple Soloists   169
  Ensemble Recording   173
  Background Vocals in Popular Music   176
Summary   177
Further Reading   178

Appendix 1: Glossary   179
Appendix 2: Power Source (Breathing) Flip Book   187
Appendix 3: Sound Source (Vocal Fold Vibration) Flip Book   191
Appendix 4: Sound Modifier (Oral Tract Area) Flip Book   195

Index   199

Preface

The last few decades of the 20th century have seen very rapid advances in personal computer technology, and this has had an impact on the working lives of many people. This has occurred at a time when significant advances in scientific knowledge in relation to voice production have also been made to the point where it is now quite straightforward to study the vocal output quantitatively on an ordinary home or office multimedia PC. Members of the next generation of singers and actors are pressing for more knowledge of the process of voice production, how best acoustic advantage can be taken of a performance space, and how to make a high quality voice recording. Underpinning all three of these highly important issues is the acoustics of voice production, the acoustics of spaces, and the basic theory and practice of recording.

This book provides an introduction to all three between two covers. Under-pinned with the basic scientific principles required to understand the key issues, it aims to offer real-world practical advice to all who work with voice, whether they are (a) on the performance stage in the theater, opera house, school classroom, lecture hall, church, conference hall, consulting room, auction house, market stall, senate, parliament, TV or radio studio, or debating chamber, (b) involved in working with the voices of others as directors, producers, coaches, pedagogues, or teachers, or (c) engaged in making voice recordings or capturing vocal performances as studio/live-sound engineers, researchers, speech and language therapists, journalists, or bedroom musicians.

The art of vocal performance can benefit from the science of voice production, spaces, and making recordings. We offer this book as a handbook to all engaged in voice work.

David M. Howard and
Damian T. Murphy
York, April 2007

For Mum and Dad who passed away during 2007
David Howard

For Helen
Damian Murphy

CHAPTER 1

Introduction

OVERALL SCOPE

Many of us use our voices regularly on a daily basis without giving a thought to routine maintenance (would you run your car this way?), any form of vocal exercise (would athletes run a race without warming up their muscles beforehand and cooling them down afterwards?), or whether our vocal output could be improved both in terms of efficiency for us as speakers and message clarity for our listeners. There appears to be an underlying tacit assumption that the voice exists and it will always be there at our disposal. While this is true, it is clear that professional voice users can achieve so much more with their voices, whether they are opera singers filling a huge auditorium singing across a very wide range of musical notes and being heard over an orchestra without amplification, or actors producing text that can be heard even when producing an apparently effortless throw-away whisper from a big stage in a large theater.

Professional voice users are trained vocally to use their voices in an acoustically efficient manner. They know some-

thing about how the voice works, and they are very aware of the acoustic environments in which they work. Some professional voice users make use of microphones to excellent effect, both on stage and in the recording studio. Some understanding of the underlying bases of how the voice works, the acoustics of spaces, and how to make a good recording will enable all speakers and singers to improve their vocal skills in their everyday professional lives, their home lives, and in on-stage vocal performance; this is the overall scope of this book.

The overall scope of this book encompasses the provision of practical help and advice to those who want to use their speaking and/or singing voices to best effect in different acoustic environments, such as classrooms, concert halls, recital rooms, opera houses, conference auditoria, theatres, churches, cathedrals, basilicas, lecture halls, debating chambers, parliament buildings, recording studios, television and radio studios, factories, auction houses, or even outside. Many professionals who use their voices on a daily basis have had no formal voice training, and they are often left struggling to cope vocally in spaces where it might be difficult to be heard and understood towards the back, or where there is a significant level of competing acoustic noise from other sources that might be outside the room itself or from others within the room. There are simple measures that can be taken to improve matters that do not involve rebuilding the space (although this might be the best plan ultimately since so many of these issues arise from poor or zero acoustic design in the first place). Others may want to make use of a microphone either to amplify their voice in order for it to be heard in a large space or to make a recording for research, archiving, or other purposes. A number of guidelines are offered relating to the use of microphones which, if followed, can result in excellent recordings that do not suffer from issues such as distortion, howl, hum, buzz, or clipping.

These suggestions are underpinned with sufficient basic science to foster a proper understanding of how the voice itself works acoustically, how sound builds up in a room, and how microphones work and can be used to best effect. There are five chapters. The first is this introduction, which covers the basic science of acoustics that is required to understand the material covered in the book as well as some of the underlying issues facing a professional or amateur vocal performer. Chapter 2 describes human voice production from a physiological and acoustic point of view, and offers some basic guidance on maintaining a healthy voice. The third chapter delves into the acoustics of spaces with a particular emphasis on how the acoustics of a space can affect speech and singing, offering advice on how one might take best advantage of the local acoustic when performing. Chapter 4 outlines the

principles for making a voice recording and includes a description of the equipment required and how to make best use of it. The fifth chapter considers the practical use of electronic amplification and the different ways in which it can help a vocal performer in practice. References and further reading are presented at the end of each chapter and a glossary of commonly found terms used in this field is provided as an appendix.

Above all, this book exists to provide practical advice for vocal performers, and each of the main chapters (2–5) ends with a section that offers practical advice for improving vocal performance. Like so many other activities in life, the best approach is probably to study one or two points of advice at a time and work with them until they become routine before moving on to others. Vocal performance is an individual and very personal skill that draws on so many aspects of our abilities, and we can only make our own individual judgment as to which aspects might serve to make overall improvements. But whatever the process adopted, any potential for even a small change to be adopted offers the possibility for an overall improvement in performance impact. Just a relatively small increase in knowledge based on the material presented in this book could result in a very large gain in the overall effectiveness of the process of communicating with one's listeners.

INTRODUCTORY ACOUSTICS

Although this book is fundamentally about the art of vocal performance, it is covering the area from a scientific viewpoint. A much deeper understanding of voice production can be gained if a multidisciplinary approach is taken, particularly when looking at performing in a space and the interaction with room acoustics and how to make a high quality recording. We believe that to cover the material in this book in a useful, solid, and unambiguous manner, the detail must be rooted in physical principles in order for the topics to make practical sense. Many of today's voice teachers and professional voice users are themselves beginning to seek a fuller understanding of what is actually going on in their vocal instrument and the effects that changes can make and why, and rigorous answers can only be given in terms of the physics that underpins voice production.

In order to do this appropriately, some essential basic scientific points are required, and that is the purpose of this section. For some, this material will already be familiar and they should skip straight to Chapter 2. However, for many voice performers, this material is worth reviewing before proceeding to later chapters. It should be noted that this can only be a brief introduction, providing revision of essential basic scientific points. Some readers may wish to pursue these matters further, and suggestions for further reading are provided at the end of the chapter.

Numbers Large and Small

As humans, we are used to dealing with numbers in everyday life, for example when using money or considering percentages. Most of the numbers encountered are typically in the range from 0 to 100, such as percentages, the number of pence in a pound, or cents in a dollar. In the world of scientific measurement, numbers are encountered that are very much larger or very much smaller than the 0–100 range, and prefixes are commonly used to allow the values themselves to be quoted in a more convenient range.

Table 1–1 lists prefixes with their multiplying factors, equivalent power of 10, and symbols that are commonly used in scientific work. Some of these are already in common usage and familiar in everyday language, such as millimeter (mm), centimeter (cm), kilometer (km), and kilogram (kg). Others are entering the language as technology develops, and examples can be found for large numbers in the computer industry and for small numbers in electronic engineering. The multiplying factor is conveniently expressed as a power of 10 as shown, which indicates the number of zeros for factors greater than 1, and one less than the number of zeros for factors smaller than one.

By way of example for large numbers, consider computer hard disk sizes which used to be quoted in kilobytes (kb), where one byte is a unit of computer data consisting of 8 binary numbers such as 10010011. As demand grows to store increasingly large amounts of computer data, particularly audio and video material, new technologies are developed to increase the available hard disk capacity. Having started being quoted in thousands of bytes (kilobytes), computer hard disk capacity moved to being quoted in millions of bytes (megabytes or Mb), and is now quoted started in thousand million bytes (gigabytes or Gb). In large research computers and computer servers, disk sizes are quoted in million million bytes (terabytes or Tb), or thousand million million bytes

Table 1–1. Prefixes, multiplying factors, equivalent powers of ten, and symbols used to make working with very large and very small numbers more convenient

Name	Multiplying Factor	Power of 10	Symbol
yocto-	0.000000000000000000000001	10^{-24}	y
zepto-	0.000000000000000000001	10^{-21}	z
atto-	0.000000000000000001	10^{-18}	a
femto-	0.000000000000001	10^{-15}	f
pico-	0.000000000001	10^{-12}	p
nano-	0.000000001	10^{-9}	n
micro-	0.000001	10^{-6}	µ
milli-	0.001	10^{-3}	m
centi-	0.01	10^{-2}	c
deci-	0.1	10^{-1}	d
kilo-	1,000	10^{3}	k
mega-	1,000,000	10^{6}	M
giga-	1,000,000,000	10^{9}	G
tera-	1,000,000,000,000	10^{12}	T
peta-	1,000,000,000,000,000	10^{15}	P
exa-	1,000,000,000,000,000,000	10^{18}	E
zetta-	1,000,000,000,000,000,000,000	10^{21}	Z
yotta-	1,000,000,000,000,000,000,000,000	10^{24}	Y

(petabytes or Pb). Information and data are always being created, and it is therefore likely that one day, storage capacity will be quoted in million million million bytes (exabytes or Eb), then thousand million million million bytes (zettabytes or Zb), and perhaps even million million million million bytes (yottabytes or Yb).

In electronic engineering, components used in circuits can have a very large range of available values. For example, a capacitor is a component whose value is measured in the unit Farads, and electronic circuits require capacitors with values in thousandths of a farad (millifarad or mf), millionths of a farad (microfarad or μf—notice the use of the Greek letter *mu* here), thousand millionths of a farad (nanofarad or nf), or million millionths of a farad (picofarad or pf).

Very large and very small numbers are needed when we want to measure natural phenomena in our world, and it is important to become familiar with the notion of dealing with values that are outside the comfortable 0–100 range. In the exploration of the acoustics of the human voice, acoustics of spaces, and how to make a recording, numbers outside this comfortable range are needed, particularly the prefixes deci-, milli-, and micro-. While this is a common concept in science, it is perhaps less commonly encountered by vocal performers and those working with the human voice.

Sound Transmission and Velocity

Changes in the weather alter the atmospheric pressure of the air around us, and these variations of high and low pressure that are seen on a weather chart typically occur over 12 hours or more. Sound is also a change in air pressure local to the source of sound, but the key difference is that the pressure changes associated with sound occur very much more rapidly, between around 20 times a second and 20,000 times a second. Such changes are known as *sound* or variations in *acoustic pressure.* It is interesting to note that our hearing system has evolved to receive acoustic pressure variations over this range of change, and it specifically excludes our hearing the pressure changes associated with the weather.

Acoustic pressure variations travel in a medium such as air in a straight line outwards from the sound source. Any medium through which sound can travel can be considered to be a series of point masses at the molecular level that are interconnected by springs to represent the forces between the molecules. A sound source sets up acoustic pressure variations, or movements of the point masses immediately adjacent to the sound source, and these movements will be transmitted to the neighboring point masses via the interconnecting springs. Figure 1–1 illustrates this for an input pulse displacement of the left-hand mass as shown. Each line in the figure is the state of the point masses after one time step, which is the time taken for the pulse to move from one mass to its neighbor. The input pulse moves the first mass to the right at the first time step, and then back to the left at the second time step as indicated. Notice that the masses themselves return to their starting position after the pulse has passed. This is a basic characteristic of sound transmission, that the molecules themselves move to transmit the acoustic pressure variation, but once this pressure variation has passed by, then they

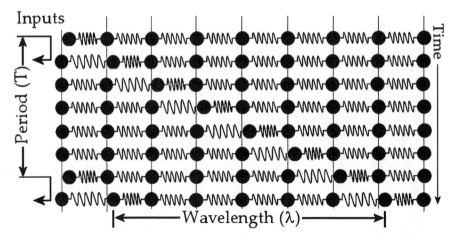

Figure 1–1. *Point mass and spring model of sound transmission in one dimension showing the transmission of two input pulses along the line of point masses with time. The distance between the repeating pulses is the wavelength (λ) and the time between them is the period (T).*

return to their starting *rest* or *equilibrium* position.

Any sound source will produce a changing pattern of pressure variation and this pattern will be radiated outwards from the source. This pattern is the *sound wave*. Notice from Figure 1–1 that for sound transmission, the point masses move in the *same* direction as the direction of travel of the sound wave; this wave motion is known as a *longitudinal wave*. A traveling wave would also be created if the point masses moved up and down in the figure because the interconnecting springs would still transmit the movement from one point mass to its neighbors (if you hold the end of a rope which is tied at the other end and move the end up and down, a wave is sent along the rope); such wave motion in known as a *transverse wave*. A transverse wave is how the strings of stringed instruments, such as a guitar, piano or violin, vibrate.

Figure 1–2 illustrates the transmission of a sound wave in two dimensions,

and it can be thought of as extending the one-dimensional set of point masses and springs (see Figure 1–1) into two dimensions to create a sheet of point masses and springs. The principle of transmission remains the same, and any acoustic pressure change at a point mass will be communicated to all its adjacent point masses that are connected to it via springs. Thus in the example illustrated in Figure 1–2, the sound pressure pulse radiates from its source (snapshot 1 in the figure) outwards in a circle from the source of sound. Notice how it is reflected from the boundaries and transmitted through the gap in the horizontal divider. Following the same principles, the thinking can be extended into three dimensions (not easy to in two dimensions on paper!), when the sound pressure changes at a point mass are communicated to all its adjacent point masses that are connected to it via springs. In three dimensions, the sound pressure wave radiates outwards spherically from the source of sound.

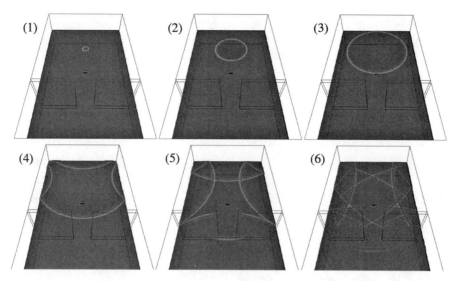

Figure 1–2. *Illustration of sound transmission in two dimensions as snapshots (1–6) showing a sequence of a pulse wave moving outwards from its source (snapshot 1).*

The transmission of pressure variations from one point outwards to other point sources via the interconnecting springs takes a finite time. Sound travels at the *velocity of sound*, or the *speed of sound*, which for air at 20° centigrade is 344 meters per second, or 344 m/s. The velocity of sound is usually denoted as C. Knowing the velocity of sound allows the time sound takes to travel a certain distance to be calculated. If a listener's ear or a microphone is 5 meters (m) from a sound source, then the time (in seconds) that sound will take to be transmitted over this distance is the distance (5 m) divided by the number of meters that sound can travel in one second (s), or its velocity (344 m/s), which is 0.0145 s. Such values look rather small, and humans prefer to deal with values that lie ideally between 1 and 100. There is no exception in acoustics, and small time values would usually be quoted in thousandths of a second, or milliseconds (ms), by multiplying the value in sec-

onds by 1000, so that 0.0145 s becomes 14.5 ms. Time values quoted in ms are common in voice analysis, because the acoustic signal changes rapidly during speech or singing.

Knowing the velocity of sound, an important relationship can be explored using Figure 1–1. A second pulse is shown in the figure occurring at a later time (recall that each line in the figure is the state of the point masses after one time step), and the time between two repeating events is known as the *period*, or *T*, as shown. The period is measured in seconds. When the second pulse is input at the left-hand side of the figure, the first pulse has traveled along the point masses and it can be seen further along to the right. The distance between the two pulses measured along the point masses is the distance between the pulses in space, and this is known as the *wavelength*, usually denoted by the Greek letter lambda (λ), as shown. The wavelength is measured in meters. Knowing that the speed of sound in air is 344 m/s enables the distance traveled by a sound pressure pulse in a given time to be calculated. In relation to Figure 1–1, the wavelength (λ) is the distance traveled during the period (T), and therefore the wavelength is equal to the speed of sound multiplied by the period (equation 1-1).

$$\lambda = C \times T \qquad (1\text{-}1)$$

The number of periods occurring in one second is known as the *frequency*, or f, and the units of frequency are *Hertz*, or *Hz*. Knowing the period, the frequency can be calculated by dividing the period into 1 to find the number of periods in one second as follows.

$$f = \frac{1}{T} \qquad (1\text{-}2)$$

This can be rearranged to give the period (T) in terms of frequency (f) as follows.

$$T = \frac{1}{f} \qquad (1\text{-}3)$$

Using this relationship between f and T given in equation 1-3, equation 1-1 can be rewritten in terms of frequency by substituting (1/f) for T as follows.

$$\lambda = \frac{C}{f} \qquad (1\text{-}4)$$

This relationship is more usually presented as follows, which involves multiplying both sides of equation 1-4 by f.

$$C = f \times \lambda \qquad (1\text{-}5)$$

It can also be used to find the frequency for a given wavelength (this will be

needed in Chapter 3) ,which involves dividing both sides of equation 1-5 by λ.

$$f = \frac{C}{\lambda} \qquad (1\text{-}6)$$

The wavelengths of different frequencies that humans can hear can be calculated using equation 1-5. The human hearing range is usually quoted as being from 20 Hz to 20 kHz (the high frequency end is reduced with age), and this can be expressed as a range of wavelengths using equation 1-4 as follows.

$$\lambda_{20\ Hz} = \frac{C}{f} = \frac{344}{20} = 17.2\ m \qquad (1\text{-}7)$$

$$\lambda_{20\ Hz} = \frac{C}{f} = \frac{344}{20,000} = \qquad (1\text{-}8)$$

$$0.0172\ m = 1.72\ cm = 17.2\ mm$$

Thus sounds that we hear have wavelengths that vary between 17 m and 17 mm. The wavelength is important in acoustic terms when considering how sound waves are affected by obstructions (such as furniture, bookcases, people, pillars, and other objects) as they travel through air. A useful rule of thumb is that when the wavelength is greater than the size of the object, the sound wave passes by as if the object is not there, and when the wavelength is less than the size of the object the sound wave is reflected by the object.

Waveforms

In order to study the nature of acoustic pressure variations, they are usually plotted as a graph of the pressure change against time, known as a *waveform*, at a particular position, for example the location of a microphone.

Examples of complete and zoomed acoustic pressure waveforms are shown in Figure 1–3 for sung versions of the vowels in *Bart* and *beat*, which exhibit regular repetitions of a pattern (upper image) and spoken versions of the consonants in *Sue* and *shoe*. Each acoustic waveform is a plot of acoustic pressure on the vertical, or Y, axis against time on the horizontal, or X, axis. The vertical axis is sometimes labeled *amplitude*, which simply means *size* of something;

in this case, amplitude would mean pressure. In general, depending on the nature of the sound source, the observed acoustic pressure variations will take one of two underlying forms: they will either exhibit a regularly repeating pattern (as for the vowels in *Bart* and *beat* shown in the upper zoomed plots in Figure 1–3) or they will not (as for the consonants in *Sue* and *shoe* shown in the lower zoomed plots in Figure 1–3). The pattern that is repeated, for example in the vowels in *Bart* and *beat*, is known as a *cycle*, and waveforms with

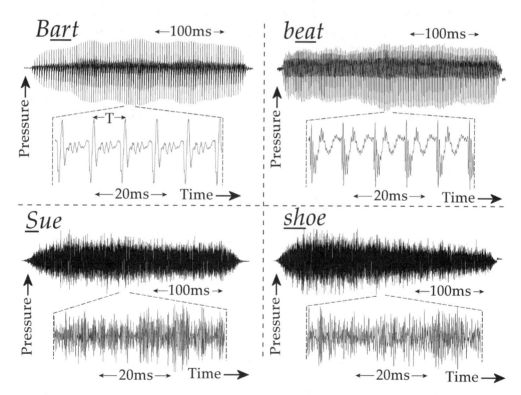

Figure 1–3. *Complete and zoomed acoustic pressure waveforms for sung versions of the vowels in* Bart *and* beat, *which exhibit regular repetitions of a pattern (upper image) and spoken versions of the consonants in* Sue *and* shoe, *which do not exhibit a regularly repeating pattern (lower). One cycle and its period, from which the fundamental frequency (f0) can be calculated (see text), are shown for each of the vowels (there are no cycles for the consonants shown here because they exhibit no regularly repeating pattern).*

repeating patterns like this are *periodic* waveforms.

When listening to periodic sounds, they have a distinct musical note, or *pitch*, associated with them. A higher pitch is perceived when the fundamental frequency (f0) is raised, or the period is lowered and there more cycles occur in one second, and vice versa. For the vowel in *Bart* plotted in Figure 1–3, the period (T) is indicated, and it can be measured as being approximately 9.0 ms. From the period, f0 can be calculated as how many cycles of 9.0 ms fit into one second (or 1 divided by 9.0 ms), which gives 111 Hz. Any waveforms, such as those for the consonants in *Sue* and *shoe* shown in the lower plot of Figure 1–3 that exhibit no repeating pattern, are *nonperiodic* (or *aperiodic*) waveforms. Nonperiodic waveforms have no cycles, no period, and no f0, and there is no strong sensation of pitch associated with them.

Sine Waves and Harmonics

The acoustic pressure waveform is a plot of the pressure variations that are transmitted from the sound source to the listener's eardrum. The difference between various sounds is manifested in the shape of the acoustic pressure waveform. For example, the two vowels shown in Figure 1–3 have periods that are very similar (compare the values for T in each case) but the shape of the repeating cycles for each vowel is very different. We hear this dissimilarity as a distinct vowel difference when listening to speech sounds, but it applies equally to the difference between two musical instruments playing the same note. For example, we can tell the difference between a flute and an oboe when they

play a note at the same pitch, and this difference is described as timbre.

The pattern of pressure variation in the acoustic waveform is specific to a particular sound. It would not be easy to describe these shape differences as a way of characterizing the acoustic distinctiveness of individual sounds. To do this, we turn to a mathematical finding that is core to many scientific disciplines, including engineering, physics, and mathematics, which notes that any periodic waveform, such as those for the vowels in *Bart* and *beat* shown in Figure 1–3, can be completely and uniquely described by a set of individual *frequency components* (or *Fourier components* after the French natural philosopher Joseph Fourier who proposed this as a theorem in the early 19th century). Each of Fourier's frequency components is a *sine wave*, and using a specific set of sine waves, a unique waveform can be completely and uniquely synthesized (the so-called *pure tone* that is produced by a struck tuning fork is a sine wave). The sine wave is therefore the building block for other periodic waveforms, and it is sometimes referred to as a *simple waveform* to distinguish it from all other periodic waveforms which are referred to as *complex periodic waveforms*.

Figure 1–4 shows a plot of a sine wave, and its key elements are labeled. The *amplitude* is the size of the excursion made by the waveform, and in practice it will have some units associated with it such as volts (electrical) or pressure (acoustic). The *period* or *cycle* is the length of the repeating part of the waveform and it can be measured between any two points that delimit that repeating part. A sinewave has positive and negative peaks, and this distance between them is known as the peak-to-peak

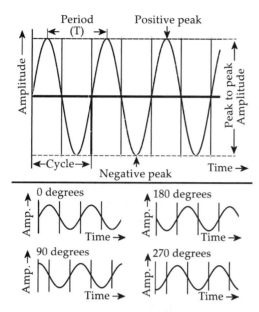

Figure 1–4. *A plot of a sine wave (simple waveform).The upper plot shows a cycle, the period, a positive peak, a negative peak, and the peak to peak amplitude. The lower plot shows phase differences, which indicate that position in time of the waveform, and this is expressed in degrees, where a change of 360 degrees is a complete cycle.*

amplitude as shown. The *phase* indicates the current position within a cycle relative to a particular point in time. Four different phases are illustrated and they are measured in degrees around a circle from 0 degrees (midpoint rising), a quarter of the way through a cycle at 90 degrees (positive peak), half way through a cycle at 180 degrees (midpoint falling), and three quarters through a cycle at 270 degrees (negative peak).

The frequency components from which a periodic waveform can be synthesized are all sine waves that have a special relationship with each other, in that their frequencies are all integer (1, 2, 3, 4, etc.) multiples of the f0 (1*f0, 2*f0,

3*f0, 4*f0, etc.). Such a set of frequency components is known as *harmonics*, and they can be referred to individually using their integer multiplier (or *harmonic number*). For example, the frequency component that is 3*f0 is the *third harmonic*, and the frequency component that is 19*f0 is the *nineteenth harmonic*. The frequency component that is 1*f0 we have already referred to as the fundamental frequency or f0, but it can also be referred to as the *first harmonic*.

By way of a quick recap, any periodic waveform is either a *simple waveform*, in which case it is a sine wave, or it is a *complex periodic waveform*, in which case it is not a sine wave, but it can be synthesized from a number of sine waves which are harmonics (integer multiples of f0).

Figure 1–5 shows a complex periodic waveform and the specific set of harmonics that are its building blocks, and Table 1–2 fully defines each harmonic. There happen in this example to be 10 harmonics (shown as the 1st to the 10th), and each is a sine wave or a simple waveform (notice that the shape of the repeating part is the same—*sinusoidal*—shape). The amplitudes (or vertical size) of each of the 10 harmonics are specific to this particular complex periodic waveform, and their relative values are given in Table 1–2. The frequencies of the harmonics are all related, by integer multiplication, to the f0 by definition, and the f0 can be found from the period of the complex waveform (see Figure 1–4). This can be confirmed by noting that the periods of the summed waveform and that of the f0 component shown in Figure 1–5 are the same. The phases are given form completeness, although they are all zero degrees; notice that each of the 10 harmonics starts by

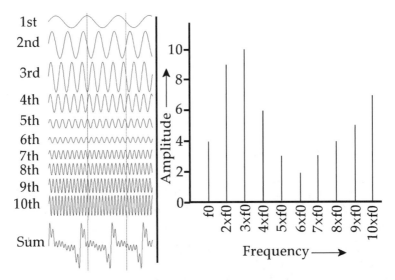

Figure 1–5. *Sample synthesis of a complex periodic waveform (sum) from 10 harmonics (left) and the representation of the 10 harmonics on a spectrum*

Table 1–2. Harmonic amplitudes, frequencies, and phases for the 10 harmonics used for the sample complex periodic waveform synthesis shown in Figure 1–3

Harmonic	1st	2nd	3rd	4th	5th	6th	7th	8th	9th	10th
Frequency	$1 \times f0$	$2 \times f0$	$3 \times f0$	$4 \times f0$	$5 \times f0$	$6 \times f0$	$7 \times f0$	$8 \times f0$	$9 \times f0$	$10 \times f0$
Amplitude	4	9	10	6	3	2	3	4	5	7
Phase (deg)	0	0	0	0	0	0	0	0	0	0

rising from its midpoint (compare with the plot for a phase of zero degrees in Figure 1–4). The resulting complex periodic waveform is synthesized by summing the values of all 10 harmonics at every point in time.

Short-Term and Long-Term Average Spectra

The harmonics are completely described by the values given in Table 1–2, which is a much more compact description than a full plot of the waveforms and their sum. Each harmonic that contributes to the sum that fully describes a complex periodic waveform is completely described by its harmonic number, amplitude, and phase. The fundamental frequency itself has to be defined also. The human ear is not sensitive to the absolute phase value of a waveform (even though it is highly sensitive to phase when it is changing), and therefore phase is usually ignored when considering a speech or singing acoustic pressure waveform. The usual way that the frequency components that make up a complex periodic waveform are represented is illustrated in the right-hand plot in Figure 1–5, which is known as a *spectrum*. This is a plot of amplitude against frequency, and a vertical line is used to represent each harmonic, and such a spectrum is sometimes referred to as a *line spectrum*. In this case, there are 10 harmonics that are equally spaced in frequency, because they are all integer multiples of f0, and the length of each vertical line shows the amplitude of each harmonic (compare with the amplitude values given in Table 1–2).

Complex nonperiodic waveforms, which have no repeating pattern (see Figure 1–3), can also be considered in terms of a unique set of sinusoidal components. However, the spectrum for a nonperiodic waveform does not have harmonics associated with it. One way of thinking about this is to consider what its f0 would be based on what is known about its waveform. F0 is directly related to the period of a periodic waveform, and f0 can be found in the case of a periodic waveform by dividing its period into one to establish how many cycles there are in one second. In the case of a nonperiodic waveform, it never repeats by definition and there are no identifiable cycles. The waveform of a nonperiodic waveform could be observed forever, and no repeating cycle would be apparent, so its period is therefore infinite. The f0 for an infinite period can still be found as one divided by the period, and one divided by infinity is zero. The f0 is therefore 0 Hz, and this is the spacing between the harmonics. The harmonics are spaced by 0 Hz, and are therefore infinitesimally close together; individual harmonics do not exist. In other words, there are components at all frequencies, and it would not be helpful to draw a vertical line for each one on the spectrum. The amplitudes of the components are therefore indicated on the spectrum as a graph showing component amplitudes against frequency. Such a spectrum for a nonperiodic waveform is known as a *continuous* spectrum, reflecting its nature as a continuous horizontal plot and differentiating it from the line spectrum for a periodic waveform.

The mathematics behind the Fourier theorem allows the spectrum to be calculated for any complex periodic or nonperiodic waveform using a computer. Figure 1–6 shows examples of spectra (plural of spectrum) for the four waveforms shown in Figure 1–3, which serves to illustrate the differences between the spectrum of a periodic waveform (the vowels in *Bart* and *beat*) and that of a nonperiodic waveform (the consonants in *Sue* and *shoe*). The spectra for the periodic waveforms exhibit clear individual components, which are the harmonics as illustrated. The amplitude of each harmonic can be measured from the spectrum, enabling the specific set of building blocks for a particular waveform to be established (see Figure 1–5). It can be seen that these two vowels have very different spectra. Note that the spectrum presented here is a plot of amplitude against frequency, but there is no analysis of phase. The phases for each harmonic are available from spectral analysis, but when working on speech and singing, phase is usually ignored because (a) humans cannot hear absolute phase differences; (b) although we can hear a rapidly changing phase, this does not occur during speech or singing (but rapidly changing phase can be synthesized electronically for sounds that might be

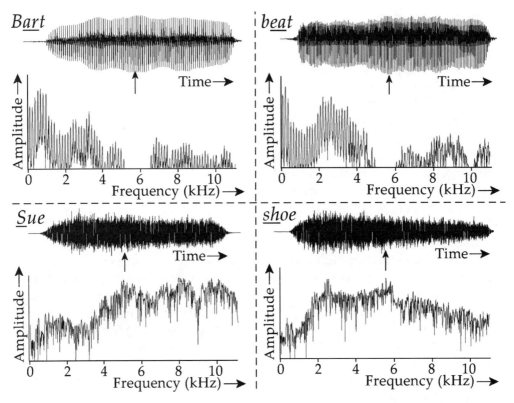

Figure 1–6. *Short-term spectra for sung versions of the vowels in* Bart *and* beat *and spoken versions of the consonants in* Sue *and* shoe, *for which waveforms are shown in Figure 1–3.*

used for music making); and (c) rapidly changing phase does not occur in natural speech or singing and therefore it plays no part in communicating the message.

The spectra for the consonants in *Sue* and *shoe* illustrate the nature of continuous spectra, which exhibit no evidence of harmonics on comparison with the spectra for the two vowels. The shape of the continuous plot is different for these two consonants; for example, the spectrum for *Sue* has more energy towards high frequency region than does the spectrum for *shoe*.

There are two types of spectra that are used in speech and singing work which are known as a *short-term spec-*

trum or a *long-term average spectrum*. The spectra shown in Figure 1–6 are short-term spectra, because they are based on an analysis of a rather short portion (20 ms) of the waveform. Short-term spectra are useful for gaining a snapshot in time at the spectrum of a sound, but if there is any noise associated with the original sound, this will contaminate the plot. One way of reducing the unwanted effects of contaminating noise on the analysis is to use a long-term average spectrum (LTAS). An LTAS takes the average of successive short-term spectra over whatever time is desired, and it is particularly useful when analyzing a sound that remains essentially static, like a sustained vowel. The effect of long-term averaging is to enhance the wanted sound itself, which is always present, while reducing the effect of unwanted noise, which will be random in nature and therefore will average towards zero.

Sample LTAS plots are given in Figure 1–7 for the complete vowel in *Bart* and the consonant in *shoe*, whose waveforms and short-term spectra are plotted in Figures 1-3 and 1-6, and for a short passage read by an adult male and a song sung by a soprano. The harmonics in the vowel are more clearly shown in the LTAS than in the short-term spectrum in this example, demonstrating the enhancing effect of averaging. However, it must be noted that this vowel was sung, and therefore its harmonics remained somewhat constant in frequency (no human can produce a completely accurate monotone!), and there remains some evidence of the harmonic structure in the LTAS. For the consonant, the LTAS plot is smoother than the plot for the short-term spectrum since some of the underlying random nature of this noise-based sound has been averaged out to leave evidence of the core spectral shape. The LTAS for the spoken passage and the song provide an indication of their overall spectral ranges, and such plots might perhaps be used to establish the working range of a specific voice in a particular speaking or singing performance situation.

Spectrograms

During speech and singing, the sounds change (otherwise nothing much would

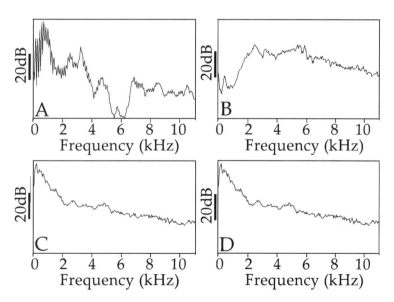

Figure 1–7. *Long-term average spectra (LTAS) for: (A) a sung version of the vowel in* Bart, *(B) a spoken version of the consonant in* shoe, *(C) a 90 s passage read by an adult male, and (D) a song sung by a soprano. Waveforms and short-term spectra for the vowel and consonant are shown in Figures 1–3 and 1–6.*

be communicated!). A short-term spectrum provides information about an individual sound, and an LTAS can provide an overall averaged spectral picture, but during speech or singing, it is the *changing* nature of the sounds being produced that is important for perceiving the message. What is required is a representation of the changing spectrum over time, and this is provided by a *spectrogram*. It is worth being aware of one potential source of confusion relating to the name *spectrogram*. The *spectrogram* is the output analysis picture from a machine or device known as a *spectrograph*. This somewhat confusing use of the suffixes *-gram* and *-graph* is a historical legacy dating from the 1940s, when the early acoustic spectral analysis machines were given the name *spectrograph*.

A spectrogram is a grayscale or color plot showing the acoustic energy present in a signal at different frequencies against time (see the diagram in the upper part of Figure 1–8). The change in frequency content of a sound over time can therefore be observed and measured from a spectrogram. There are two types of spectrogram commonly used for the analysis of speech and singing, known as *wide-band* and *narrow-band spectrograms*. The difference between them relates to the way the analysis itself is carried out, and it can be illustrated by considering the spectrograms presented in Figure 1–8 for the word *eye* spoken on a falling pitch and then sung by an adult male.

The first characteristic to note about the spectrograms is that energy is shown as the darkness of grayscale marking in

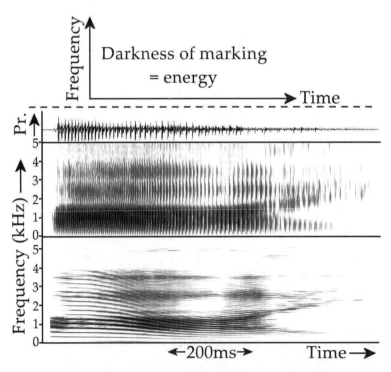

Figure 1–8. *Sketch to illustrate the axes of a spectrogram, speech pressure waveform, and wide-band and narrow-band spectrograms of eye spoken on a falling pitch and then sung by an adult male.*

these examples. While this is at one level done to enable the production of a non-color page in this book, there is a far more fundamental reason for not using color when interpreting spectrograms. A color spectrogram will make use of different colors to represent different energy level ranges. For example, different colors might be used to indicate different acoustic energy level ranges as follows: white (80–100%), yellow (60–80%), orange (40–60%), red (20–40%), and blue (0–20%). This will produce a very colorful picture which might indeed be considered far more visually attractive than a grayscale version. However, it is potentially misleading. The eye is drawn to those places in the spectrogram where the color changes—perhaps a yellow-orange boundary strikes the eye in particular—suggesting that there is a degree of importance associated with this area of the spectrogram. But all this apparent boundary represents is those places where the energy level happens to change between arbitrary spectrogram plotting levels, in this example between yellow (60–80%) and orange (40–60%). The use of a continuously changing scale, such as a grayscale or a graded change in just one color, removes any possibility of misleading the eye because no such boundaries will be visible on the spectrogram (see Figure 1–8).

The most obvious global difference between the wide-band and narrow-band spectrograms is in their underlying structure. The wide-band and narrow-band spectrograms are based mainly on vertical and horizontal lines, respectively. This betrays the underlying analysis accuracy of each spectrogram. The wide-band spectrogram provides a good time analysis, shown by vertical lines or *striations*, which denote discrete positions along the time (X) axis. The narrow-band spectrogram provides a good frequency analysis, shown by horizontal lines or *harmonics* in the case of a periodic sound or frequency *components* in the case of a nonperiodic sound, which denote discrete positions along the time (X) axis.

In practice, both wide-band and narrow-band spectrograms are used for speech and singing analysis, offering greater accuracy for time and frequency measurements, respectively. In the example spectrograms shown in Figure 1–8, it can be seen that there are clearly visible changes occurring in both for the spoken word *eye*. The harmonics are clearly visible in the narrow-band spectrogram as the horizontal lines. Recalling that the lowest, or first, harmonic is f0 and all the others are integer multiples (1, 2, 3, 4 . . .) of f0, harmonics will always be equally spaced at any given point in time. The word *eye* in the figure was spoken on a falling pitch, and the harmonics are all falling in frequency. Given that they are equally spaced by definition (the spacing is always f0 because f0 is the difference between any two adjacent harmonics such as the 7th and the 6th), notice that on the narrow-band spectrogram, they move closer together as the pitch falls. Conversely, they would move further apart for a rising pitch.

The wide-band spectrogram also exhibits the falling pitch, but now it is in relation to the spacing between the vertical lines or striations. Each striation indicates the cycle of the acoustic pressure waveform, so as the pitch falls, the period of each cycle becomes larger (less cycles per second as the pitch falls and therefore a lower f0), and the distance between the striations becomes greater. It would not be feasible to make a measurement of the period from the inter-striation distance without zooming in considerably. If f0 measurements are to be made from a spectrogram, the narrow-band version is usually used, and improved accuracy is obtained if the frequency of a high harmonic is measured and the answer is divided by the harmonic number. For example, if the frequency of the 10th harmonic is measured, the answer would be divided by 10. Other key features with respect to the acoustics of speech production are shown on the spectrograms, and these are detailed and discussed in Chapter 2.

Decibels

When sound intensity levels are being measured, the values are quoted using *decibels*, or *dB*. Their origin goes back to Alexander Graham Bell, who investigated how the human hearing system perceives changes in the loudness of sounds when the sound intensity level is changed. Loudness does not change on the basis of a linear change, which would mean that the addition of a fixed sound intensity value would produce a fixed increase in loudness; rather, loudness exhibits step changes for fixed ratio changes in sound intensity (for example, a doubling in sound intensity always produces the same perceived change in loudness). Mathematically, such a change is described using a logarithmic scale, which exhibits the property that a particular ratio change has a fixed distance along a logarithmic scale. Logarithmic scales turn out to be the basis not only of our perception of loudness. They also reflect our perception of frequency, musical intervals, smell, vision, and touch.

Bell proposed converting sound intensity to a logarithmic scale so that quoted values reflect how perceived

loudness changes. In order to do this, a given measured value of sound intensity has to be compared with some reference in order to form a ratio from which to take a logarithm. The softest sound intensity level that can, on average, just be heard was found (its value is 1 picowatt per square meter, or 10^{-12} Wm^{-2}). The scale that Bell proposed was called the *Bel* scale, and values were calculated by taking the base 10 logarithm of the ratio of the measured value of intensity to the reference value of intensity as follows.

$$Bel = \log_{10}\left\{\frac{I_{measured}}{I_{reference}}\right\} \quad (1-9)$$

It is worth noting that when the measured intensity is equal to the reference intensity, the intensity ratio is 1. The logarithm of 1 is 0, so a value of 0 Bels indicates that the *value is equal to the reference value*, and *not* that it equals 0. The maximum sound level that humans can hear without causing pain was found to be around 10 watts per square meter, or 10 Wm^{-2}. Its value in Bels is found by substituting this value into equation 1-9 along with the reference (10^{-12} Wm^{-2}), to give 13 Bels as follows.

$$Bel_{10Wm-2} = \log_{10}\left\{\frac{10}{10^{12}}\right\} = \quad (1-10)$$
$$\log_{10}\{10 \times 10^{12}\} = \log_{10}\{10^{13}\} = 13 \text{ Bels}$$

As humans, we generally prefer to deal with numerical values between around 0 and 100, so the Bel scale, which ranged from 0 Bels to 13 Bels, was multiplied by 10 and therefore called the decibel, or dB, with a range between 0 dB and 130 dB.

The shorthand for decibel based on sound intensity level is dB(SIL), and it is found as follows.

$$dB(SIL) = 10 \times \log_{10}\left\{\frac{I_{measured}}{I_{reference}}\right\} \quad (1\text{-}11)$$

If a decibel value for a sound pressure level, or dB(SPL), is being measured, for example when using a sound pressure level, or SPL, meter, then the logarithm is multiplied by 20 rather than 10, as shown in equation 1-12. This is because intensity is proportional to the square of pressure. Doubling the logarithm is mathematically equivalent to squaring the ratio, which changes the multiplication factor from 10 to 20. The reference value for dB calculations using acoustic pressure is 20 microPascals, or 20 µPa (see Table 1–1).

$$dB(SPL) = 20 \times \log_{10}\left\{\frac{P_{measured}}{P_{reference}}\right\} \quad (1\text{-}12)$$

Table 1–3 lists typical dB(SPL) values found for everyday sounds by way of an approximate guide to what a particular sound level in dB is equivalent to. The reference level is defined as the threshold of hearing, the sound level that on average can only just be heard, and by definition of the decibel, this is 0 dB. At the highest sound levels, the sensation of hearing changes to one of feeling and then to one of pain. This occurs at around 120 dB and 130 dB, respectively, but these values are based on measurements made some decades ago. It is now known that exposing the human hearing system to such high levels for extremely short periods of time, less than the time required to make the measurement, can cause permanent hearing damage. Table 1–3 shows that the range of sound pressure levels that can be heard by the human hearing varies between 20 microPascals, or 20 µPa, and 20 million microPascals, or 20 Pa (notice that the

million cancels out the micro—see Table 1–1). This illustrates another very important aspect of using a logarithmic scale; it compresses huge ranges of numbers into a much easier to appreciate range, which in this case is 0 to 120.

Another key feature of the dB scale is that a change of a fixed number of dB represents a fixed multiplication of the measured value; this is a basic property of the logarithm. For example, it is often useful to know the dB change that is equivalent to a doubling or halving of sound intensity, and this can be found from equation 1-11 by substituting 2 or 0.5 for the intensity ratio as follows.

$$dB_{\text{sound intensity doubling}} = \quad (1\text{-}13)$$
$$10 \times \log_{10}\{2\} =$$
$$10 \times 0.301 = 3.01\ dB$$

$$dB_{\text{sound intensity halving}} = \quad (1\text{-}14)$$
$$10 \times \log_{10}\{0.5\} =$$
$$10 \times (-0.301) = -3.01\ dB$$

The dB change that is equivalent to a doubling in sound intensity is therefore 3.01 dB, and that for a halving of sound intensity is −3.01 dB.

When working with sound pressure levels, the dB change for a doubling or a halving is also a useful figure to be aware of, and these can be found from equation 1-12 by substituting 2 or 0.5 for the pressure ratio as follows.

$$dB_{\text{sound pressure doubling}} = \quad (1\text{-}15)$$
$$20 \times \log_{10}\{2\} =$$
$$20 \times 0.301 = 6.02\ dB$$

$$dB_{\text{sound pressure halving}} = \quad (1\text{-}16)$$
$$20 \times \log_{10}\{0.5\} =$$
$$20 \times (0.301) = -0.602\ dB$$

Table 1–3. Typical sound pressure levels in decibels, or dB(SPL) values, along with the equivalent sound pressure levels in microPascals (μPa) and Pascals (Pa), and typical sounds for each level listed.

Pressure (μPa)	Pressure (Pa) ($P_{measured}$)	dB(SPL) $20 \times \log_{10}\left\{\dfrac{P_{measured}}{P_{reference}}\right\}$	Typical Sound
200,000,000	200	140	Jet take off at 10 m
63,200,000	63.2	130	Threshold of pain—jet taking off at 40 m
20,000,000	20.0	120	Threshold of feeling
6,320,000	6.32	110	Peak level: opera singer fortissimo (*ff*) at 1 m
2,000,000	2.00	100	Shout or yell at 1 m
632,000	0.632	90	Heavy diesel engine (high throttle) at 1 m
200,000	0.200	80	Vacuum cleaner at 1 m
63,200	0.0632	70	Opera singer singing piano (*p*) at 1 m
20,000	0.0200	60	Conversational speech at 1 m
6,320	0.00632	50	Background level in office
2,000	0.00200	40	Whispered speech at 1 m
632	0.000632	30	Background level in a quiet home
200	0.000200	20	Quiet in a well-designed performance hall
63.2	0.0000632	10	Wilderness on a still day
20.0	0.0000200	0	Threshold of hearing—complete silence

Notice that the dB change that is equivalent to a doubling or halving in sound pressure is twice that for a doubling or halving in sound intensity, because the multiplying factor is 20 rather than 10.

In summary, a few key points are worth noting about decibels.

1. The decibel is a measurement that is *relative* to a reference.

2. 0 dB does not mean a signal level is zero; it has the same value as the reference.
3. The dB scale compresses a huge range of Pa values into a convenient range.
4. A doubling in sound intensity is an increase of approximately 3 dB.
5. A halving in sound intensity is an increase of approximately –3 dB.
6. A doubling in sound pressure is an increase of approximately 6 dB.
7. A halving in sound pressure is an increase of approximately –6 dB.

THE PERFORMER'S VOICE

Everyone who makes use of his voice in daily life is a vocal performer. However, for the majority, the voice is simply a bodily function that is there to be used. Most employers make demands on the voices of their employees to a greater or lesser degree, and again, voice production is essentially taken for granted. Voice complaints are commonplace among voice users, whereas voice production knowledge is sparse. One purpose of this book is to provide some practical tips relating to healthy voice production that have the potential to benefit all voice users. In addition, the descriptions relating to the acoustics of spaces and how to use them to best vocal advantage (Chapter 3) provide a basis for a greater understanding of the voice in context as well as practical guidance.

All professional vocal performers are aware to a greater or lesser degree of their voices, and most will have had professional vocal training (just occasionally, a natural voice emerges that works very effectively without training inter-vention). The majority of vocal training that is available makes use of an oral culture in which technique is handed down from teacher to pupil as an oral tradition from one generation to the next. This process is a highly qualitative one, and one which typically involves prior vocal knowledge, experience from the teacher's own performance career, and imagery. Imagery appears to be a technique that is common and fundamental to the work of the professional voice teacher, and it often occurs in the form of concepts, or *psychological hooks*, offered as instructions, such as: *"Sing on the point of the yawn,"* or *"Sing as if smelling a flower,"* or *"Sing as if through the top of your head."* Psychological hooks such as these are used to encourage changes in, for example, posture or breathing, in order to achieve an appropriate (to the ears of the teacher) vocal output. There is no doubt that such psychological hooks can enable pupils to enhance their voice production skills, but few, if any, of the instructions offered as such hooks bear any relation to the physical reality of the process of voice production.

SUMMARY

Many students and teachers are now searching for descriptions of the voice production process that bear a one-to-one relationship to changes that need to be made to the physical instrument, the body of the performer. The last quarter of the 20th century has seen huge advances in knowledge of voice production in terms both of the instrument itself and the acoustic output. In addition, many of the scientific analyses that were only possible in a speech science laboratory a few decades ago are now available on a standard multimedia PC. Many teachers are realizing this and wanting to make use of scientific analyses in their teaching activities to enhance the learning experience through the use of (a) descriptions based on physical reality, (b) real-time displays of measured parameters relating to voice production, and (c) as a means of tracking vocal change over time.

It is these aspects that in part have prompted the writing of this book, and in particular Chapter 2, which provides an introduction to the acoustics of voice production. A proper understanding of voice acoustics is absolutely basic to being able to interpret appropriately the results from scientific measurements, and to make use of them in practice. It must be remembered that this area brings together the disciplines of art with those of science, and we all have much to learn as we delve into a discipline other than one that is core to our own experiences. This book brings science as an offering to the art of vocal production. It must, however, be made quite clear that it is not being suggested that a scientific approach could ever take over the process of professional voice teaching. Any scientific approach will always only be another tool in the armory of a professional voice teacher that is there to be used when the teacher deems it appropriate, in much the same way as a mirror or a piano might be used.

No scientific approach will ever replace a professional teacher for the development of artistic performance. There are aspects of vocal training and education where the judgment of another human will always be required and where the use of a scientific measurement is highly unlikely to offer any advantage, such as stagecraft, performing musically, working with accompanists, working with conductors, working with directors, communicating with the audience, gesture, posture, ornamentation, etc. The use of scientific measurement to speed up the process of achieving some of the basics has the potential to free up more lesson time for these essential and often somewhat neglected building blocks of performance.

During any vocal performance, the sound reaches the ears of the listeners via the local environment, which will impart its own acoustic signature on that sound. Performers and directors who are aware of these effects can take steps to make best use of the acoustics of the space to enhance the overall result. Chapter 3 describes the way in which the acoustics of the local environment affects the voice on its journey from performer to listener, and offers a number of practical tips to maximize the overall experience for both performer and listener. This material is probably even more important for those whose everyday employment takes them into environments that are poorly suited to vocal performance (such as many school classrooms, some hotel seminar and conference rooms, some hospital consulting rooms, some interview rooms, some rehearsal rooms, and some offices), where there was probably little or no acoustic design input to the building of the space, and where, for many, long periods of time are spent engaged in speaking or singing.

The other aspect of vocal performance that is covered in this book is that of voice recording and electronic ampli- fication of the voice. There are many who want to make recordings in which they sing to backing tracks that they have recorded using a computer. There are those who are engaged in profes- sional scientific research on the voice for whom high quality recordings are the essential starting point. Many voice per- formers make use of microphones and electronic amplification both to enhance the sound heard by the listeners and to allow them to hear their own voice at an appropriate level. Selecting the most appropriate equipment and setting it up appropriately for the space in which it is being used can make a huge difference to the overall performance or recording result, enhance the confidence of the performer, and raise the appreciation level of the listeners.

In the context of this book then, the vocal performer is anyone who uses his voice on a regular basis. He may have had no vocal training, he may have no awareness of which parts of his body he uses when speaking or singing, but he is likely to be aware when his voice is not functioning normally or when it is a struggle to speak or sing in some rooms compared to others. Something can be done about most of this for those willing to invest the time to find out more. These pages are offered as a resource for all performers.

FURTHER READING

Introductory Acoustics

Baken, R. J. (1987). *Clinical measurement of speech and voice*. London: Taylor and Francis.

Borden, G. J., & Harris, K. S. (1980). *Speech science primer*. Baltimore: Williams & Wilkins.

Hall, D. E. (1980). *Musical acoustics—An intro- duction*. Belmont CA: Wadsworth.

Harris, T., Harris, S., Rubin, J. S., & Howard, D. M. (1998). *The voice clinic handbook*. London: Whurr.

Howard, D. M., & Angus, J. A. S. (2006). *Acoustics and psychoacoustics* (3rd ed.). Oxford, UK: Focal Press.

Rosen, S., & Howell, P. (1990). *Signals and systems for speech and hearing*. London: Academic Press.

Rossing, T. D. (1982). *The science of sound*. New York: Addison-Wesley.

Speaks, C. E. (1992). *Introduction to sound*. San Diego, CA: Singular.

Sundberg, J. (1989). *The science of musical sounds*. San Diego, CA: Academic Press.

The Performer's Voice

Dejonkere, P. H., Hirano, M., & Sundberg, J. (1995). *Vibrato*. San Diego, CA: Singular.

Potter, J. (1998). *Vocal authority*. Cambridge, UK: Cambridge University Press.

Potter, J. (2001). *The Cambridge companion to singing*. Cambridge, UK: Cambridge University Press.

CHAPTER 2

The Human Voice

INTRODUCTION

One of the first things that a newborn baby does is to cry in a wonderfully loud, natural, unimpeded, and open manner. This most basic activity provides a means of communicating with those around to request essential needs for living and growing up. A baby is born with the ability to make sounds using the voice production instrument, and during the early years of childhood, the sounds produced develop into the language in local use through listening, imitating, and observation of the responses obtained.

The cry of a newborn baby is acoustically efficient, free, and very well projected. It can be heard at a considerable distance and the instrument itself is working in a highly efficient manner. However, this natural formula for playing the vocal instrument is rarely left unhindered and therefore does not last. A child's developing use of the vocal instrument is conditioned by parental and peer response, which so often serves to inhibit efficient voice production and dampen vocal performance confidence

as the child is told for example, to "pipe down," "stop making such a noise," "stop shouting as we cannot hear ourselves think," "only speak when spoken to," "be seen and not heard," "make a noise quietly," or "stop singing" Depending on the severity with which such instructions are given, a typical response might be some degree of clamming up in terms of vocal output. This is likely to be accompanied by and in part due to increased muscular stress, especially in the neck and shoulder regions, which is in itself a common habit associated with 21st century living that is fundamental to poor vocal health. Coupled with the psychological result of being told by parents and peers that a loud vocal output executed in a free and efficient manner is not routinely acceptable in daily life, the clamming up and stressed response becomes normal vocal habit for many.

Unpacking these and other aspects of less efficient, unnatural, and clammed up vocal output is a key step to healthy voice production and being able to project the voice efficiently in a babylike fashion. Some knowledge of the voice production process in terms of its anatomy and physiology, as well as the acoustics of both the voice production process and rooms, can greatly enhance progress in healthy voice development. Singing and speech make use of the same vocal instrument, and the underlying anatomical, physiological, and acoustic principles involved are common to both activities.

This chapter provides an introduction to the anatomy and physiology of the human vocal instrument and then focuses on the resulting acoustic output. The presentation concentrates only on those aspects that are vital for a proper and fully informed understanding of the basics of human voice production in the context of vocal health and efficiency, as well as vocal production in different acoustic environments and making a successful voice recording. The singing as well as the speaking voice is considered, and the chapter ends with a number of everyday tactics that can be employed to maintain the voice in a healthy state.

VOICE PRODUCTION

This section describes the main parts of the human body that are involved in voice production, whether speaking or singing. In order to produce a sound with any system, whether an acoustic musical instrument, an environmental noise, the call of an animal, or an electronically synthesized sound, three essential features must exist:

- power source
- sound source
- sound modifiers

Human voice production during speech or singing is no exception, and therefore it will be described here in terms of the *power source, sound source,* and *sound modifiers*. During sung notes, these correspond anatomically to the action of the *lungs,* the *vocal folds,* and the *vocal tract,* respectively. These are illustrated in Figure 2–1, which also shows an equivalent mechanical model, indicating with double-ended arrows those parts that can be moved during speech or singing. The relevant anatomical and physiological detail of the power source, sound source, and sound modifiers are described below in terms of their function during voice production, the acoustic output, and useful tips for maintaining a healthy voice.

Power Source in Voice Production

The power source in a musical instrument might, for example, be the bow moving across the string of a stringed instrument; a finger plucking a string on a stringed instrument; the lungs blowing air into a woodwind or brass instrument; a finger striking the key of a piano or harpsichord; the electrical power supply of an electronic instrument; the blower of a pipe organ; or the stick or beater striking a percussion instrument. For the human voice, the power source is the flow of air from the lungs via the throat and mouth and/or nose during exhalation. Indeed, it is the same power source used when playing woodwind and brass musical instruments.

Breathing is a natural function which is automatic and basic to life itself. While the airways are open and the lungs maintain a higher air pressure than the

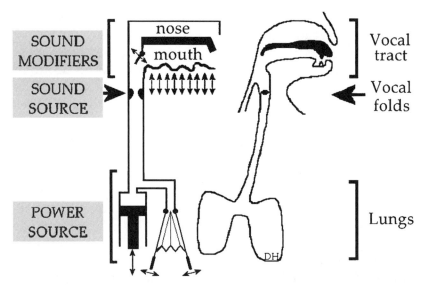

Figure 2–1. *An overview of the human vocal instrument when the vocal folds are vibrating during either singing or speech in terms of its three main constituent parts: power source (lungs), sound source (vocal fold vibration), and sound modifiers (vocal tract spaces). The anatomical equivalent is shown on the right and an equivalent simple mechanical model on the left.*

atmospheric pressure outside the body, air flow is sustained from the lungs to the outside world via the mouth and/or nose. When lung air pressure is lower than the atmospheric pressure of the local environment, air flow is sustained to the lungs from the outside world. This is the basic physics behind how we breathe. We change the air pressure in the lungs relative to atmospheric pressure when we breathe. On breathing in when singing or speaking in a healthy manner, air is drawn into the lungs by enlarging the lung spaces through muscular action, which is equivalent to pulling the piston in Figure 2–1 downwards and the bellows outwards. This produces a lung pressure that is lower than external atmospheric pressure (same quantity of air now occupying a larger volume results in a reduction in

pressure), and air will flow into the lungs (providing the upper airway is open). When we breathe out, through muscular action we contract the lungs (equivalent to pushing the piston in Figure 2–1 upwards and/or the bellows inwards), thus producing a lung pressure that is higher than external atmospheric pressure (same quantity of air now occupying a smaller volume results in an increase in pressure) and air flows out from the lungs (providing the upper airway is open).

The lungs themselves are such that if they were removed from the body they would shrink greatly in size. Each lung can in this respect be considered, albeit rather crudely, as being somewhat similar to a balloon. However, there is a fundamental difference between a lung and a balloon in terms of inflation and deflation. The lungs are supported externally within the rib cage and from below by the diaphragm so that they can be physically enlarged to suck air in. Breathing in and out is a result of lung expansion and contraction, which is achieved by the actions of muscles as illustrated in Figure 2–2. First, there is a group of muscles that can move the rib cage by expanding it outwards or contracting it inwards. The muscles that join with and control the size of the rib cage during breathing are known as the intercostals. The inspiratory intercostals expand the rib cage and are therefore used when breathing in, and the expiratory intercostals contract the size of the

rib cage and hence can be used when breathing out.

Second, there is the action of the diaphragm which is attached to the lungs. The diaphragm is bowed upwards below the lungs when it is relaxed, as shown in Figure 2–2. When it is contracted, it becomes shorter and its shape flatter, expanding the lungs by pulling them downwards (like a piston in a cylinder). In addition, the lower rib cage is opened outwards (rather like a blacksmith's bellows). The lower part of Figure 2–2 illustrates an ideal breathing sequence for which there is a flip book version in Appendix 2. The diaphragm sits over the abdominal wall, and since

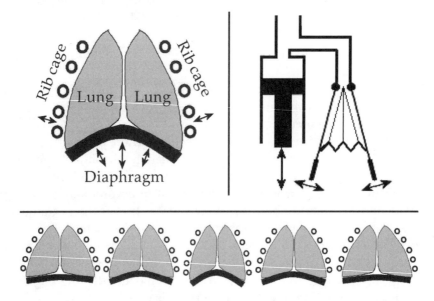

Figure 2–2. *An overview of breathing during singing and speech showing how the lungs can be expanded and contracted using the rib cage and/or the diaphragm, alongside the power source part of the equivalent mechanical model shown in Figure 2–1. The double-ended arrows indicate movement which can increase and decrease the volume of the lungs, and the model indicates the piston- and bellows-like nature of lung action during breathing. The lower part of the figure shows an idealized breathing sequence for which a flip book version can be found in Appendix 2.*

the volume of the abdomen itself and its contents cannot be altered appreciably, any diaphragm contraction serves to push down on the abdomen, which causes the abdominal wall to bulge outwards and air to enter the lungs (if the airway is open). The diaphragm is relaxed following contraction, and it returns to its rest position and air is expelled from the lungs (if the airway is open). Note that the lungs are not empty when the diaphragm is at its rest position; they can be further compressed to enable longer phrases to be spoken or sung. Abdominal wall expansion and contraction are readily observed externally in the region of the navel, and this provides a useful indicator of diaphragmatic breathing.

In summary, during breathing the following muscles can be used:

■ breathing in: the inspiratory intercostals and/or the diaphragm
■ breathing out: the expiratory intercostals and/or the abdominals

Notice that these are the muscles we *can* use to breathe and stay alive. The upper chest region can also become engaged in the process of breathing, as observed for example during rapid panting. However, healthy voice use requires that the upper body (chest, shoulder, and neck region) remains relaxed in order that the neck and larynx are relaxed and under no excessive strain. This precludes the use of the upper chest region for breathing when engaged in healthy voice production, so the predominant muscles used for breathing are the diaphragm, intercostals, and abdominals. Many voice teachers refer to the notion of *support* or *supported breathing*, which provides a practical form of instruction, something

that might be termed a *psychological hook*, to focus the mind of the performer on controlling (or supporting) the lungs from below.

Sound Source in Voice Production

The sound source during sung notes results from the vibration of the vocal folds in the larynx. In this book, the term *vocal folds* is used to describe the vibrating elements in the larynx, because it describes most appropriately the physical nature of the vibrating structures. In medical circles, the vocal folds are more usually referred to as the *vocal cords*, which has its origins in what Manuel Garcia saw when he looked down the throat with his 45 degree mirror (probably seeing the light reflecting from the upper edges of each vocal fold, which would have appeared to be string- or cordlike). The media and other sources often use the term *vocal chords*, which is a misnomer, although one quick-thinking York student justified the use of this term in his submitted work by arguing that the observed shape of each vocal fold from above was a *chord* of a circle!

When a sung note is produced and the vocal folds vibrate, the resulting sound is heard as having a *pitch*. Such sounds are described as being *voiced*, because they involve vocal fold vibration in the larynx or *voice box*. Not all of the sounds used in spoken communication are voiced and produced as a result of the vibrating vocal folds, however. There are *unvoiced* or *nonvoiced* sounds in speech that result from air being forced past a narrow constriction in the mouth or oral cavity, such as the final consonants in the words *pass*, *stiff*, and *pitch*.

Finally, there is a third sound source used in voice production which is a mixture of the voiced and voiceless source, when the vocal folds vibrate and air is forced past a constriction, and this sound source is termed *mixed*. The final consonants in the words *fez*, *pave*, and *badge* have a sound source that is mixed.

In summary then, there are three sound sources used in speech and singing as follows:

- **voiceless** (involving air being forced past a constriction in the vocal tract)
- **voiced** (involving vocal fold vibration)
- **mixed** (involving voiced and voiceless sound sources)

In terms of vocal training, almost all effort relating to the sound source is devoted to voiced sounds and the vibrating vocal folds. This is particularly true for singing training, since a basic requirement is to gain a much wider pitch range than is used for normal speech.

A voiceless sound source involves a narrow constriction somewhere in the vocal tract, for example between the upper teeth and lower lip during the production of the final consonant in *stiff*. If air flows sufficiently fast through the constriction, it becomes *turbulent* and a noiselike sound is produced. Such sounds are known phonetically as *fricatives*. The occurrence of a noiselike sound when air flow is rapid enough can be confirmed by forming a constriction between the upper teeth and lower lip in preparation for producing an *f* sound and adjusting the air flow from slow to fast while listening to the acoustic result. Voiceless sounds have no definite pitch associated with them; you cannot sing notes on them—try singing the final consonants in *pass*, *stiff*, and *pitch*. The production of

a voiceless sound source is learned as speech is acquired, and unless there is some speech-related issue about inappropriate positioning of the constriction within the vocal tract, which would be dealt with by a speech and language therapist, nothing additional is needed for the professional voice user. The remainder of this section therefore concentrates on the voiced sound source.

The voiced sound source results from the vibration of the vocal folds in the larynx. The larynx is situated in the neck, and it can be located by moving the side of an index finger gently up and down the front of the neck to find the prominence on the thyroid cartilage, known as the *Adam's apple*, which can be observed in the illustration of the larynx shown in Figure 2–3. The Adam's apple is usually more obvious and clearly visible for men than it is for women, because the adult male larynx is approximately twice as large in its linear dimensions. If the side of the index finger is placed in contact with the neck on the prominence of the Adam's apple while swallowing, a vertical movement of the whole larynx structure can be felt. This demonstrates that the larynx is supported by muscles in the neck; it is not held rigidly in position.

Vocal fold vibration for a voiced sound source is initiated by bringing the vocal folds closer together horizontally—a movement known as vocal fold *adduction*. Voiced sounds are normally produced when exhaling (breathing out). As air is expelled past the gap between the adducted folds (this gap is known as the *glottis*), the velocity of air flow must increase because the airway is narrower. One physical consequence of increasing the velocity of air flow due to a constriction is that the push or pressure that it exerts on the sides of the tube is reduced. This is known as the *Bernoulli effect*. It should be noted that it is possible to produce voiced sounds when inhaling (breathing in). This is something that can occur automatically when one is communicating in a high state of panic, shock, or fright to allow communication to take place continuously, even when breathing in. Producing a voiced sound source when inhaling is also part of some vocal warm-up/cool-down exercises.

The Bernoulli effect is also the principle upon which aircraft fly. Aircraft wings are shaped as shown in the upper part of Figure 2–4. Air flowing across the upper surface has further to travel due to the upward curve in the wing profile, and therefore less pressure is exerted downward on the upper surface of the wing compared to the pressure exerted upward on the lower surface, resulting in *lift*, as illustrated. The Bernoulli effect as it relates to the closure of the vocal folds can be demonstrated by blowing across a sheet of paper held at the end nearest the lips, as shown in the lower part of Figure 2–4. The sheet will rise up (note the similarity in shape between the curved sheet and the upper surface of the aircraft wing) due to the Bernoulli effect.

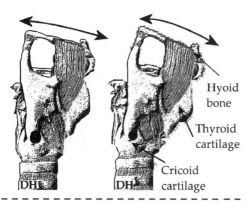

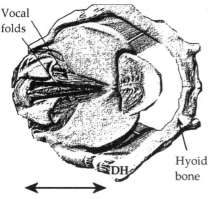

Figure 2–3. *Illustration of the tilting mechanism of the larynx, which enables the length of the vocal folds to be altered and thereby the fundamental frequency of their vibration and the perceived pitch. The upper panel shows a side view to illustrate how the thyroid cartilage hinges on the cricoid cartilage (marked with the black circle). The lower panel looks down on the larynx, revealing the vocal folds, which are stretched and relaxed as a direct result of the tilting mechanism.*

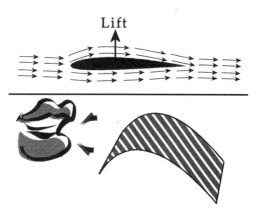

Figure 2–4. *Illustration of the Bernoulli principle as it relates to how aircraft fly based on the profile of their wings (upper), and a demonstration of the Bernoulli principle by blowing across a sheet of paper held as shown at the end nearest the lips (lower).*

During vocal fold vibration, air flows between the adducted vocal folds through the narrowed glottis, where the air velocity increases with the consequential decrease in pressure on the sides of the tube (the vocal folds themselves), as described by the Bernoulli effect. The reduction in pressure on the vocal folds acts to move them towards each other, in a manner somewhat analogous to the lift on an airplane wing. The result of moving closer together is that the glottis is narrowed even more, the air flow velocity increases, the pressure exerted on the vocal folds (tube walls) reduces, and the force pulling the folds together increases. The vocal folds therefore accelerate towards each other as they get closer together, until finally they meet at the midline with a "snap" as the glottis closes.

From the closed position, the vocal folds will open because they have closed off the air flow from the lungs, where air is under pressure. In addition, the folds have a natural tendency to return to their rest/starting position—each vocal fold can be thought of as behaving like an oscillating pendulum. Each vocal fold will move like a pendulum past its rest, or *equilibrium*, position, on to its fully open configuration, and back towards its equilibrium position. The Bernoulli effect again comes into play and the cycle repeats, resulting in sustained oscillation. As the vocal folds vibrate, their lower edges will meet and part before their upper edges, since the folds have depth as well as width (see Figure 2–5), and the Bernoulli effect acts on their lower edges first, due to the direction of air flow. A flip book version can be found in Appendix 3.

In speech and singing, the pitch of the voice is always changing. Even in

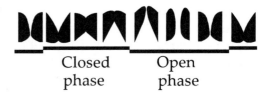

Closed phase   Open phase

Figure 2–5. *Illustration of the sequence of vibration of the vocal folds viewed from the front (a flip book version of this figure is available in Appendix 3). Notice that opening and closing start from the lower margins and move upwards.*

singing when one attempts to sing a steady note, there will be small changes in pitch. During speech, changes in voice pitch are the "tune" of the language, or *intonation* pattern. English uses intonation to signify, for example, whether or not one is uttering a statement or a question as in the following: *"That train is late!"* and *"That train is late?"* Singers change the pitch to alter the note they are singing, and to tune their voices with other singers or any accompanying musical instrument(s). In speech, pitch tends to be thought of in terms of a changing contour, whereas in singing, pitch relates to discrete notes.

The pitch of the vibrating vocal folds can be changed by altering their mass, tension, and/or elasticity; this is described by the *myoelastic aerodynamic theory of vocal fold vibration* (see Van den Berg [1958] in the further reading list for more details). Increasing the mass, reducing the tension, or making the elasticity smaller will have the effect of lowering the pitch, and vice versa. In practice, the mass can be changed by holding a portion of each vocal fold immobile, which means that their vibrating masses are reduced and the pitch will rise. The vocal folds are supported within the larynx within a hinged structure, as illustrated in Figure 2–3, in such a way that the folds can be stretched and released, raising and lowering their f0, respectively.

Sound Modifiers in Voice Production

The acoustic characteristics of a sound will be modified by the spaces through which it passes in much the same way as the sound of the voice varies in different rooms and buildings. In the case of speech and singing, the sound modifiers are the spaces through which the sound source passes to emerge from the between the lips and/or nostrils of the speaker or singer. It is the shape of these spaces that serves to modify acoustically the output from the sound source. There are two spaces that make up the vocal tract:

■ **the oral cavity** (the space between the glottis and the lips)

■ **the nasal cavity** (the space between the velum and the nostrils, or the nose)

The main way in which the shape of the oral cavity (mouth and pharynx in Figure 2–6) can be altered is by moving the tongue, jaw, and lips. Such moving parts are known as the *articulators*, and those that can be moved when speaking or singing are illustrated in Figure 2–6 with double-ended arrows on the equivalent mechanical model of the sound modifiers.

The main articulators serve to alter the shape of the mouth, and the main ways in which this can be achieved in speech and singing are by varying the height of the jaw, the position of the lips between being rounded (as in the vowel in *boo*) and spread (as in the vowel in *bee*), and/or by changing the shape of the tongue by increasing the constriction between it and the hard palate using its

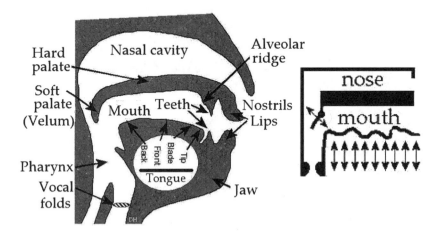

Figure 2–6. *The human vocal tract showing the main parts associated with voice production (left) alongside the sound source and sound modifier equivalent mechanical model (right), shown in Figure 2–1. The parts that can be moved are indicated by double-ended arrows on the mechanical model and their names can be found by referring to the vocal tract (left).*

tip, blade, front, or back. The nose is rather different because its shape cannot be altered. It is used in voice production for sounds such as the final consonants in *boom, bean,* and *bring,* the so called *nasal* consonants in English. The nose is engaged by changing the position of the *soft palate* or *velum,* which works as a valve to allow sound to pass through the nose or not, depending on whether it is lowered or raised, respectively (see the mechanical model in Figure 2–6). It is possible to feel the action of the velum if a hum is produced that is broken up by forming but not releasing a *b* (the first consonant in *boo*); one might write this as *mmmbmmmbmmmb.* "Not releasing a *b*" sound means not opening the lips—let it revert to the hum. It should be possible to feel the action of the velum as it is raised when the *b* is formed (to shut the nose off from the airstream), and lowered for the hum (to allow air to flow through the nose and out via the nostrils).

The minimum set of sounds required to distinguish the words of a language are those that are uniquely in the words of that language. For example, the English words *ton, done, shun, son, gun, run, won, nun, fun* indicate that the initial consonant sounds are unique phonemes for English, since exchanging them in this context produces different meaningful words. Similarly, the vowel sounds that distinguish the words *bat, bit, but, bet, boat, bait, bite, bought, beat, boot, Bert,* and *Bart* are also phonemes of English. It turns out that English has 24 consonants and 20 vowels (a total of 44 phonemes) when its unique sounds are considered, which is very different from the 5 vowels and 21 consonants (a total of 26 letters) that exist in the alphabet used when writing words; the correspondence

between the phonemes used to indicate how a word is spoken and how the word is spelt is rarely one-to-one.

The articulation of the phonemes in English would be described by phoneticians in terms of three descriptors: *voice, place,* and *manner,* which indicate whether the vocal folds vibrate or not (voice), where (place), and how (manner) the sound is produced. Table 2–1 lists the 44 phonemes of English using the SAMPA (Speech Assessment Methodologies Phonetic Alphabet) transcription system introduced by John Wells in 1989. The SAMPA system is used here because it makes use only of characters that are available on a standard computer keyboard using ordinary fonts. For each phoneme, an example word (from the world of yachting) is provided along with its SAMPA transcription, and for the consonants, their voice, place, and manner labels are provided, which are described in the next sections.

Voice

The voice label indicates whether or not the vocal folds vibrate during the production of the phoneme, which is described as being either *voiced* (V+) because the vocal folds vibrate or *voiceless* (V–) because they do not. A quick check to confirm whether the vocal folds vibrate while producing a sound can be made by either (a) putting hands over the ears and listening for a loud buzzing sound, (b) trying to sing the sound, or (c) feeling either side of the throat gently near the level of the Adam's apple for vibration. A number of English phonemes differ only by voice including the initial consonants in *Sue* and *zoo, fire* and *via, chew* and *Jew, pan* and *ban, ton* and *done,* as well as

Table 2–1. The 24 consonants and 20 vowel sounds in English with their SAMPA symbols (Sym.), example words (Word), and SAMPA (see Wells, 1989, in the reading list) transcription (Trans.). The voice, place, and manner descriptions are listed for the consonants

ENGLISH CONSONANTS

Sym.	Word	Trans.	Voice	Place	Manner
p	rope	/r@Up/	V–	bilabial	plosive
b	buoy	/bOI/	V+	bilabial	plosive
t	tide	/taId/	V–	alveolar	plosive
d	deck	/dEk/	V+	alveolar	plosive
k	cabin	/k{bIn/	V–	velar	plosive
g	galley	/g{li/	V+	velar	plosive
T	thwart	/TwOt/	V–	dental	fricative
D	weather	/wED@/	V+	dental	fricative
f	fog	/fQg/	V–	labio-dental	fricative
v	rung	/rVN/	V+	labio-dental	fricative
s	sea	/si/	V–	alveolar	fricative
z	zenith	/zEnIT/	V+	alveolar	fricative
S	ship	/SIp/	V–	palato-alveolar	fricative
Z	treasure	/trEZ@/	V+	palato-alveolar	fricative
h	heeling	/hilIN/	V–	glottal	fricative
tS	chain	/tSeIn/	V–	palato-alveolar	affricate
dZ	jibe	/dZaIb/	V+	palato-alveolar	affricate
m	mast	/mAst/	V+	bilabial	nasal
n	main	/meIn/	V+	alveolar	nasal
N	rigging	/rIgIN/	V+	velar	nasal
w	winch	/wIntS/	V+	bilabial	semivowel
r	rain	/reIn/	V+	alveolar	semivowel
l	lee	/li/	V+	alveolar	semivowel
j	yacht	/jQt/	V+	palatal	semivowel

ENGLISH VOWELS

Sym.	Word	Trans.
i	neap	/nip/
I	jib	/dZIb/
E	red	/rEd/
{	anchor	/{Nk@/
A	hard	/hAd/
Q	locker	/lQk@/
O	port	/pOt/
U	foot	/fUt/
u	food	/fud/
V	rudder	/rVd@/
3	stern	/st3n/
@	tiller	/tIl@/
eI	weigh	/weI/
aI	light	/laIt/
OI	oilskin	/OIlskIn/
@U	row	/r@U/
aU	bow	/baU/
I@	pier	/pI@/
E@	fare	/fE@/
U@	fuel	/fU@l/

cot and *got*. In each of these examples, the first of the pair is voiceless and the second is voiced. Table 2–1 shows the voice label for each English consonant.

Place

The place of articulation describes where in the vocal tract there is either a complete closure or vocal tract narrowing. The main places of articulation used for English consonants are shown in Figure 2–7 and are listed in Table 2–1. The *bilabial* sounds /p/, /b/, and /m/ involve contact between the lips. The *labio-dental* sounds /f/ and /v/ result from contact between the lower lip and the upper teeth. *Dental* articulation is used for the sounds /T/ and /D/, which use contact between the tongue tip and the upper teeth. The *alveolar* sounds are /t/, /d/, /n/, /l/, /s/, and /z/, for which the tongue tip or blade makes

contact with the alveolar ridge. The /r/ sound is *post-alveolar* because it is usually produced with tongue contact further back along the hard palate than for the alveolar sounds. There is close approximation between the front of the tongue and the area between the alveolar ridge and hard palate for /S/, /Z/, /tS/, /dZ/, and /j/, which are therefore known as *palato-alveolar*. For /k/, /g/, and /N/, the back of the tongue makes contact with the soft palate or velum and their place is described as *velar*. The sound /h/ is produced with a close approximation of the vocal folds, and its place is known as *glottal* (the space between the vocal folds is the glottis).

The vowel sounds in British English include both those that remain steady throughout (/i/, /I/, /E/, /{/, /A/, /Q/, /O/, /U/, /u/, /V/, /3/, and /@/), which are known as *monophthongs*, and those that change from one vowel to another during their production (/eI/, /aI/, /OI/, /@U/, /aU/, /I@/, /E@/, and /U@/), which are known as *diphthongs*. The production of monophthongs is described in terms of four elements: (a) how *close* or *open* the constriction is between the closest part of the tongue to the roof of the mouth, (b) whether it is the *front*, *center*, or *back* of the tongue which is making that constriction, (c) whether the lips are *rounded* or *unrounded*, and (d) whether the vowel is *nasalized*.

Traditionally, vowels are shown on a *vowel quadrilateral*, which shows the position of each vowel by indicating the position of the highest point of the tongue. The vowel quadrilateral for the English monophthongs is shown in Figure 2–8, along with an indication of the position of the quadrilateral itself in relation to tongue position in the mouth.

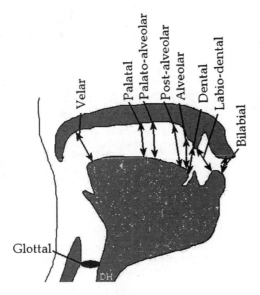

Figure 2–7. *The places of articulation used for English consonants.*

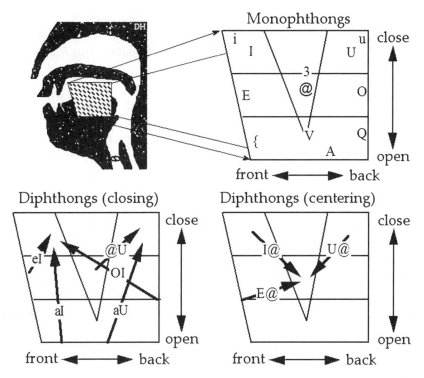

Figure 2–8. *The approximate position of the vowel quadrilateral within the vocal tract (upper left) with vowel quadrilateral plots of English monophthongs (upper right), closing diphthongs (lower left), and centering diphthongs (lower right) plotted on vowel quadrilaterals. SAMPA (Wells, 1989) symbols are used throughout.*

The vertical and horizontal axes are open/close and front/back, respectively. Lip rounding can be externally observed. The full description for the vowel /i/ is front, close, and unrounded, while /u/ is back, close, and rounded, and /{/ is front, open, and unrounded.

Any vowel can become nasalized when the velum is lowered and the nasal cavity is coupled to the oral cavity. This happens when there is a nasal consonant either before or after the vowel, and the velum is either still lowered after the nasal consonant, or lowered in preparation for the nasal consonant. A nasalized vowel is sometimes described as

sounding *hollow* when compared to its non-nasalized counterpart.

Diphthongs are vowels which do not remain steady; rather, there is a change from one monophthong to another. This can be readily appreciated in Figure 2–8 where the traditional representation of each diphthong is shown as an arrow from the first to second monophthong, which provides a representation of the associated movement of the highest part of the tongue during their production. For example, the diphthong /aI/ (*eye*) involves a glide between the monophthongs /a/ and /I/, and the diphthong /I@/ (*ear*) glides between /I/ and /@/.

Depending on their endpoint, English diphthongs are described as either *centering* (moving towards /U/ or /I/) or *closing* (moving towards /@/).

Manner

The *manner* of articulation indicates *how* the sound is articulated, and the manner for the English consonants is listed in Table 2–1. Two groups of sounds involve a complete closure. The first group (/p/ /b/ /t/ /d/ /k/ /g/) involves a sudden release of air that has been trapped in the vocal tract during a complete tract closure with the soft palate raised. These sounds are known as *plosives* (because the sound is somewhat akin to an explosion) or *stops* (because air flow is stopped in the vocal tract during their production). The time during which the air cannot flow from the vocal tract is known as the hold stage of the plosive, and during the hold stage, the air pressure in the tract builds up towards lung air pressure. When the constriction is removed (the *release* stage of the plosive), the "explosion" of this built-up pressure is released. The second group (/m/ /n/ /N/) contains the *nasal* consonants because the soft palate is lowered to allow air to escape via the nostrils during their production. The nasals involve a complete closure in the mouth, but that air pressure does not build up because the nasal airway is always open. Notice that their places of articulation match those of the plosives.

Other sounds involve a partial closure or a narrow constriction. One group (/f/ /v/ /T/ /D/ /s/ /z/ /S/ /Z/) involves the formation of a narrow gap somewhere in the vocal tract, through which air is forced to the point where its flow becomes turbulent, which causes sound to be produced. The sound produced is noiselike (for example, noise is heard if the lips are held very close together but with a tiny gap and air is blown out of the mouth rapidly). The sounds in this group of consonants are known as *fricatives,* because the noiselike sound that is made during their production is known as *frication.* The two consonants, /tS/ and dZ/, are each a plosive followed by a fricative, and they exist as phonemes in their own right because they are members of the minimum set of sounds required to distinguish the words of the English language. They have double symbols to represent them as a plosive followed by a fricative, and they are known as *affricates.* The last four consonants (/w/ /r/ /l/ /j/) are known as *semivowels* because, although they are produced in a similar way to the vowels, they are members of the minimum set of sounds required to distinguish the words of the English language and they appear in positions in words where consonants are found (consider their positions in words such as *you, zoo, woo, right, light, bight, white*). The vowels do not have special manner labels since the label *vowel* describes how they are articulated.

ACOUSTICS OF THE VOCAL OUTPUT

Power Source and Sound Source

The main function of the power source is not to create an acoustic output, but the process of breathing in and out can produce sounds which are often audible. The sound of breathing is part of the vocal output, serving to punctuate speech or singing, and as an indicator to some degree of the physical state of the speaker and singer, for example, gasping if they are out of breath or rapid harsh breaths if they are angry and/or stressed. The breath sound is a result of air flowing rapidly through a tube in which there is a constriction, and this usually occurs at the narrowed glottis. It is perfectly possible to breathe in or out inaudibly, which involves either slowing the rate of air flow or reducing the constriction, but this is sometimes not possible in the time available, depending on the context of what is being said or sung.

To recap the earlier discussion, there are three sound sources used in speech and singing as follows:

■ **voiceless** (involving air being forced past a constriction in the vocal tract)
■ **voiced** (involving vocal fold vibration)
■ **mixed** (involving voiced and voiceless sound sources)

The voiceless sound source has no musical pitch associated with it (try singing /s/ or /f/), and this means that the acoustic pressure variation associated with such sounds does not repeat, or appears visually to be random. This is illustrated in the upper left plot in Figure 2–9, which shows an idealized voiceless sound source. It can be seen that there is no repeating pattern in its waveform, and therefore its frequency spectrum is *nonharmonic* or *continuous* (see Chapter 1), and in particular, the continuous spectrum

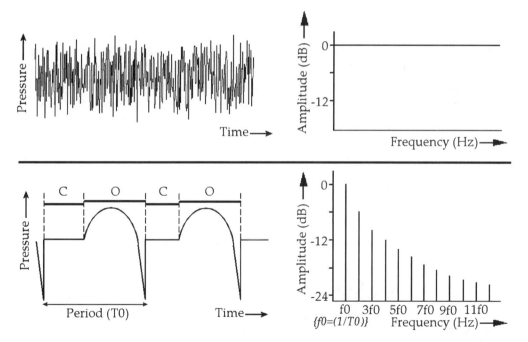

Figure 2–9. *Idealized acoustic pressure sound source waveforms (left) and spectra (right) for voiceless (upper) and voiced (lower) speech sounds. For the voiced sound source (lower left), the closed (C) and open (O) phases of the vocal fold vibratory cycle and the period of the pressure waveform are indicated. Note that the fundamental frequency (f0) is equal to the reciprocal of the period, or {f0=(1/T0)}.*

for the sound source in voiceless sounds is flat; that is, all frequency components exist with the same amplitude. Using light as an analogy, such a sound is called *white noise* on the basis that white light consists of an equal amount of all colors.

The voiced sound source has a musical pitch (a tune can be sung on a vowel), and a pitch is perceived when the acoustic pressure consists of a pattern of vibration that repeats regularly, or is *periodic*. The lower plot in Figure 2–9 shows an idealized voice sound source, and the repeating pattern can be clearly seen. The pattern that repeats represents a single cycle of vocal fold vibration, and the time taken for one cycle (the *period*) is indicated on the figure as T0. The fundamental frequency (f0) can be found from T0 as the number of cycles that occur in one second [or $f0 = (1/T0)$]. Therefore the greater the f0 value, the shorter the period (more cycles occur in one second), and the higher will be the perceived pitch. The typical spectrum for the voiced sound source is harmonic (see Chapter 1), consisting of frequency components at integer $(1, 2, 3, 4 \ldots)$ multiples of f0 (f0, 2f0, 3f0, 4f0, 5f0 . . .) as indicated in the figure. On average in speech, the height or *amplitude* of the harmonics reduces by 12 dB with each octave rise in frequency as shown in the figure. This feature of the spectrum is usually described as a *spectral slope of −12 dB per octave* (see Chapter 1). By way of comparison, the spectral slope of the voiceless sound source, which is flat, could be described as a *spectral slope of 0 dB per octave*. During singing, the spectral slope can vary depending on, for example, style, musical dynamic or loudness, or emotion.

The sound source for a mixed sound source is a combination of the voiceless and voiced sound sources. However, the voiceless sound source is not active all the time, since there is no air flow present when the vocal folds are in contact, because its path from the lungs is shut off. The voiceless component therefore switches between being on and off during each cycle of vocal fold vibration, and the voiceless element is therefore described as being *pulsed*.

As noted previously, the majority of speech and singing teaching in relation to the sound source is devoted to voiced sounds. This is particularly true for singing, given the basic need to develop a much wider pitch range than is used for normal speech, and the remainder of this section is therefore devoted to aspects of the voiced sound source.

During voiced speech or singing, the vibrating vocal folds open and close usually in a regular fashion. Every instant of vocal fold closure produces a pulse of sound energy into the vocal tract. This can be thought of as being rather like a hand clap, which also produces a short pulse of sound energy (a hand clap also results from two masses—the hands—coming together until they impact together, rather like each collision of the vocal folds). During voiced speech or a sung note, vocal fold vibration is essentially regular, producing a repeating pattern of acoustic pressure into the vocal tract (see the plots for voiced sound sources in Figure 2–9). The number of cycles of this pattern (closures of the vocal folds) per second is the f0 of the resulting sound, which relates directly to the pitch that is perceived. Figure 2–10 shows the approximate ranges of f0 that are used in speech and

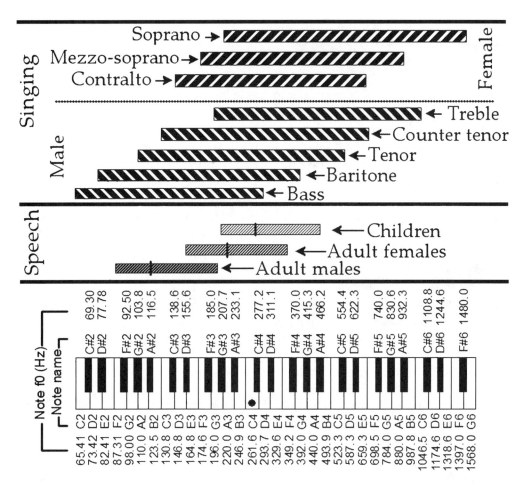

Figure 2–10. *Approximate f0 ranges in speech and singing set alongside a piano keyboard with equal tempered f0 values referenced to the international tuning standard: A4 (440 Hz).*

singing, and for reference, these are set alongside a piano keyboard with f0 values for each note, referenced to the international tuning standard of the A above middle C (usually notated as A4) being 440 Hz. It can be seen that f0 ranges in speech are considerably smaller than those used in singing. The average speaking f0 range is around 13 semitones (just over an octave), whereas for singing, the average f0 range is around 29 to 36 semitones (or 2.5 to 3 octaves).

The f0 value indicates how many vocal fold cycles occur in 1 second, and it is worthwhile noting that speech and singing can involve a very large number of closures over the course of a working day (speech) or a performance (singing). Clearly the vocal folds of adult females and children will vibrate more numerous times than those of adult males, given that they vibrate at higher values.

For example, the vocal folds of an adult female teacher using her speaking voice in the classroom could well vibrate more than *one million times in each working day*. This figure is calculated by assuming (a) an average f0 of 200 Hz, (b) an average of 6 hours' speaking time in a working day (or $6 \times 60 \times 60 = 21{,}600$ seconds), and (c) that on average, speech is voiced (as opposed to being unvoiced or there being silence) 25% of the time. These estimates result in 1,080,000 vocal fold vibrations in one day ($200 \times 21{,}600 \times 0.25 = 1{,}080{,}000$). It is little surprise that teachers suffer the most voice problems in today's society and typically are the largest client group attending for ENT (ear-nose-throat) consultations.

For a singing example, consider a soprano singing an operatic aria lasting *just 5 minutes*; her vocal folds might vibrate *over 150,000 times*. This figure is calculated by assuming (a) an arbitrary average note pitch of D5 (f0 = 587 Hz; see Figure 2–10), (b) that the aria lasts 5 minutes or $5 \times 60 = 300$ seconds), and (c) that the sung sound is pitched for 90% of the time. These estimates result in 158,490 vocal fold vibrations in a 5-minute soprano aria ($300 \times 587 \times 0.9 = 158{,}490$).

In speech and sometimes in singing, the output sound can vary in terms of its voice quality. Voice quality relates to the way in which the vocal folds vibrate, and it covers not only the normal speaking voice but also some effects used in singing and pathological voices. Four voice qualities are usually associated with normal speech voice production:

- modal (or normal)
- breathy
- falsetto
- creak (or fry)

Differences in the way the vocal folds vibrate can be monitored non-invasively using an electrolaryngograph to monitor vocal fold vibration electrically. This is achieved via two electrodes that are placed externally on the neck at larynx level, and which connect the neck to a high frequency electronic circuit whose current flow varies depending on whether the vocal folds are in contact or apart. Figure 2–11 shows the acoustic pressure waveform and the electrolaryngograph output waveform, or *Lx*, for the four

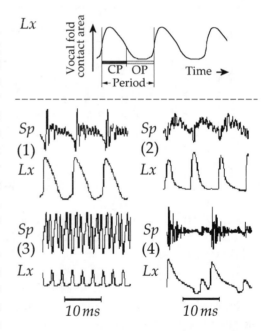

Figure 2–11. *Idealized Lx waveform (upper) showing its period, the open phase when the vocal folds are apart (OP), and the closed phase when the vocal folds are in contact (CP). Larynx closed quotient (CQ) is found as the percentage of each cycle for which the vocal folds are in contact (CQ = [[CP/period] × 100]%). Speech pressure (Sp) and electrolaryngograph output waveform (Lx) for modal (1), breathy (2), falsetto (3), and creak (4) voice qualities.*

voice qualities. The Lx waveform represents increasing vocal fold contact area (vertically upwards) against time; the steeper the Lx upward-going vertical slope the more rapid is the vocal fold closure.

Modal voice is the most commonly used voice quality in everyday speech. The full body of each vocal fold is in motion, and the folds meet at the glottal midline as they vibrate symmetrically with each other. The glottis is usually fully closed when they are in contact. The Lx output has steep upward-going vertical slopes, which indicate that there are rapid vocal fold closures. A greater level of acoustic pressure excitation to the vocal tract at high frequencies results from more rapid vocal fold closures, and this can be observed in the Sp waveform which has steep vertical variations associated with it (high frequency variations have more cycles "packed in" within a given time and their rises and falls are therefore more rapid).

During breathy voice the glottis does not fully close when the vocal folds collide, and a small gap remains through which air can escape. Although the electrolaryngograph monitors vocal fold contact, it cannot indicate whether or not the vocal folds are fully or partly closed, so the Lx output is not indicative of this aspect of breathy voice. The vocal folds remain apart (glottis open) for longer in each cycle, which is shown by the shorter vocal fold contact peaks in the Lx output. The vocal fold closures are not as rapid as in modal voice, and the consequence of this can be seen on the Sp waveform, which does not exhibit the large peak at closure that can be seen for the modal voice example. The resulting sound is noiselike due to continuous air flow through a narrow constriction (recall the description in the Introduction of this chapter of fricatives which also have air flowing through a narrow constriction) and therefore described as being breathy. Breathy voice is particularly common in the speech of adult females, and it is also, for example, typically associated with a voice that is more alluring.

Falsetto voice is occasionally used to enable high pitches to be reached during speech. The period of the Sp and Lx waveforms for falsetto are considerably shorter than those for the modal and breathy voice qualities, and therefore its f0 is higher [recall that f0 = (1/period)]. A significant portion of each vocal fold is held firmly so that it cannot vibrate, thereby reducing the mass of the vibrating portion. The contact area is therefore also reduced, and this results in a smaller amplitude Lx waveform. This reduced mass results in a higher f0 of vibration (the strings for high notes on a violin are thinner than those for the low notes), and the laryngeal hinging mechanism can still be used to vary the f0, but now it is over a higher range.

Creaky voice sounds low and rather broken up in pitch. The vocal folds are relaxed and they vibrate at a low frequency, often with more than one closure per cycle. The example Lx waveform for creaky voice exhibits two closures per cycle, a large one followed by a small one. The f0 is not always particularly steady, and the voice quality is low in pitch and it can sound somewhat rough.

One key parameter that can be derived from the Lx output is larynx closed quotient, or *CQ*. This is defined as the percentage of each vocal fold cycle for which the folds are in contact, and it is measured as illustrated in the upper plot of Figure 2–11 by finding the percentage of each cycle that is the closed phase (CP) as follows:

$$CQ = \left(\left(\frac{CP}{period}\right) \times 100\right)\% \qquad (2.1)$$

CQ has been found to change with f0 and with singing experience and/or singing training. CQ results are usually plotted as a function of f0, and Figure 2–12 summarizes the change in CQ with f0 for adult males, adult females, and children. For adult males, CQ remains relatively constant with f0, but increases with singing training/experience. For adult females, CQ is not constant as f0 changes, but its pattern of variation changes with singing training/experience such that the most highly trained exhibit higher CQ with higher f0 values. For children (girls and boys whose voices have not transformed), the variation follows a variation of CQ with f0 that is most similar to that for adult females. The CQ variation with f0 for boys follows the pattern exhibited for adult males after voice transformation.

A key finding is a tendency for an increase in CQ with singing training/experience. Three suggestions have been offered by Howard (1995) to explain this.

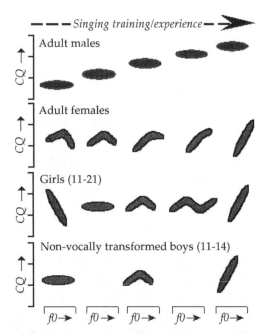

Figure 2–12. *Larynx closed quotient variation for adult males, adult females, and children with singing training/experience. Note. The data are from "Towards the quantification of vocal efficiency," by D. M. Howard, G. A. Lindsey, and B. Allen, 1990, Journal of Voice, 4(3), pp. 205–212; "Variation of electrolaryngographically derived closed quotient for trained and untrained adult singers," by D. M. Howard, 1995, Journal of Voice, 9(2), pp. 163–172; "Electrolaryngographically derived voice source changes of child and adolescent singers," by C. A. Barlow and D. M. Howard, 2005, Logopedics Phoniatrics Vocology, 30(3/4), pp. 147–157.*

1. Trained singers can sing longer notes on one breath.
   (*A longer CQ means that less lung air is used in each cycle.*)
2. Trained singers sound less breathy than untrained singers.
   (*A longer CQ equates to a shorter open phase so there is less time in each cycle for air to escape through the open vocal folds.*)
3. The voice is more acoustically efficient as more acoustic energy reaches the listener.
   (*A longer CQ means that there is less time in each cycle during which acoustic energy can "escape" to the lungs via the open glottis, from where it is lost to the outside world—an effect known as subglottal damping.*)

The Sound Modifiers

The acoustic properties of the sound modifiers are described with reference first to vowels and diphthongs, and then to manner, or *how* the sound is produced. Differences relating to the place, or *where* in the vocal tract the sound is produced, are accounted for as required.

The sound modifiers are the spaces through which the output from the sound source has to pass to reach the outside world. The sound modifiers consist of the oral cavity and, if the velum is lowered, the nasal cavity. The acoustic effect of the sound modifiers is to alter the amplitudes of the acoustic pressure components of the sound source. Idealized voiceless and voiced sound source waveforms and spectra are shown in Figure 2–9. This acoustic modification is based on the volume and shape of the sound modifiers. Only the oral cavity can be changed in volume by moving the articulators; the nasal cavity is essentially fixed in its shape. The nasal cavity contributes to the sound modification process when it is connected with the oral cavity by a lowered velum. The key acoustic principle used to describe the effect of the sound modifiers on the sound source is *resonance*.

Resonance is a natural property of physical systems, and it relates to how a system responds to an input. In particular, resonance relates to particular frequencies which are *preferred* by the system and are allowed through with little or no effect on their amplitude, as opposed to other frequencies that are reduced in amplitude as they pass through the system. The resonant properties of a system are usually plotted as a graph that indicates how a system will respond to all frequencies, a *frequency response curve*.

In the case of voice production, the resonant characteristics of the vocal tract determine how the spectrum of the sound source is modified before it arrives at the ears of the listener. The vocal tract frequency response curve contains a number of preferred or resonant frequencies which appear as peaks in the vocal tract frequency response curve. These peaks are known as *formants*, and the frequency at which the peak occurs is known as a *formant frequency*.

Vowels

The acoustics of monophthongs is described first and then that of diphthongs. Figure 2–13 shows idealized vocal tract response curves for the vowels in *Bart* (/A/) and *beat* (/i/). In each case, three *resonant peaks*, *preferred frequencies*, or *formants* are identified in the response plot of the sound modifiers. The formants are numbered in order of ascending frequency as indicated in the figure: first formant (F1), second formant (F2), and third formant (F3). In theory, a vocal tract frequency response curve contains many formants, but since their amplitudes reduce with increasing center frequency, it is rare that more than six formants can be identified for spoken or sung sounds. When considering the acoustic properties of voice production, it is usually the lower three formants (F1, F2, F3) that are considered, since these vary with the changed articulations used for different speech sounds. The higher formants (F4, F5, F6) tend to relate more to the specific shapes of fixed parts of an individual's vocal tract, thereby having the potential to contribute towards an idiosyncratic acoustic signature.

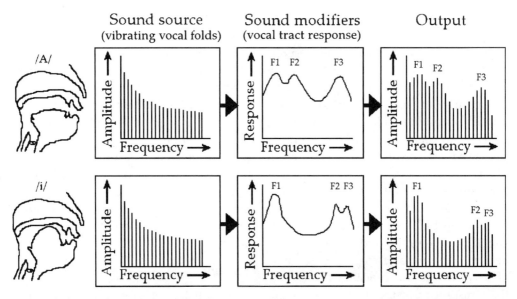

Figure 2–13. *Idealized vocal tract configurations, voiced sound source, frequency responses, and output spectra for the vowels in Bart or /A/ (upper) and beat or /i/ (lower). The positions of the first three formants (F1, F2, F3) are shown.*

Vowels are usually voiced in speech (otherwise they would be whispered) and always voiced in singing, and Figure 2–13 shows an idealized spectrum of a voiced sound source and the resulting output spectrum for each of the two vowels. The output results from the harmonics of the voice source having their amplitudes changed by the sound modifier (vocal tract) response curve, rather like superimposing the response curve onto the sound source spectrum. The formant peaks in the response curve are still visible in the output spectrum as indicated in the figure, so the perceptual system has access to the formant frequencies to enable vowel identification. It is important to note that the formant frequency itself, the peak in the sound modifier (vocal tract) response curve, is *not* available accurately from the output spectrum. The only energy in the output spectrum occurs at the frequencies of the

harmonics (integer multiples of f0) of the voice source as shown in Figure 2–13. When vowels are spoken or sung at high pitches, the harmonics are further apart since f0 is larger, and this can make identification of the formant peaks difficult in speech and impossible for high notes in singing (this is discussed further below).

For the two vowels shown in Figure 2–13, the front of the tongue is in a high position during /i/, whereas the tongue is lowered and the jaw is more open for /A/. The resulting formant frequencies are quite different due to these articulation differences. The relative positions of the formant frequencies with respect to each other are important for the perception of vowels, and it can be seen that the vowel /i/ relative to the vowel /A/ has a low F1, high F2, and high F3. A classical set of average frequencies for the first, second, and third formants published by

Peterson and Barney in 1952 is presented in Table 2–2 for men, women, and children for a selection of vowels.

The frequencies of the first and second formants for any vowel bear an interesting relationship with the position of the vowel on the vowel quadrilateral (see Figure 2–8). The variation in the frequency of F1 from low to high is equivalent on the quadrilateral to changes along the close (low F1) to open (high F1) axis. Changes in the frequency of F2 from low to high are equivalent to variation along the back (low F2) to front (high F2) axis. Monophthongs are vowels that are produced with an articulation gesture which remains essentially static, and their formants stay relatively steady in frequency. Diphthongs are vowels which are produced with an articulation change from one monophthong to another (as indicated by their SAMPA symbols and the arrows on the quadrilateral in Figure 2–8), and their formant frequencies change from those for the initial to the final monophthong over approximately 200–250 ms, or one fifth to one quarter of a second. Appendix 4 provides a flip book for oral tract shape changes during the diphthong /aI/ as in *right*.

Plosives

Acoustically, there are three significant aspects to plosives, each of which has the potential to play a part in the perception process. The first is the frequency properties of the burst, usually described as the *center frequency of the burst*; the second is the way the formants change as

Table 2–2. Average first, second, and third formant frequencies in Hz for men, women, and children for a selection of vowels indicated using SAMPA symbols

Vowel	Men F1	Men F2	Men F3	Women F1	Women F2	Women F3	Children F1	Children F2	Children F3
/i/	270	2300	3000	300	2800	3300	370	3200	3700
/I/	400	2000	2550	430	2500	3100	530	2750	3600
/E/	530	1850	2500	600	2350	3000	700	2600	3550
/{/	660	1700	2400	860	2050	2850	1000	2300	3300
/A/	730	1100	2450	850	1200	2800	1030	1350	3200
/O/	570	850	2400	590	900	2700	680	1050	3200
/U/	440	1000	2250	470	1150	2700	560	1400	3300
/u/	300	850	2250	370	950	2650	430	1150	3250
/V/	640	1200	2400	760	1400	2800	850	1600	3350
/3/	490	1350	1700	500	1650	1950	560	1650	2150

Source: From "Control Methods Used in a Study of the Vowels," by G. E. Peterson and H. L. Barney (1952), *The Journal of the Acoustical Society of America, 24*, pp. 175–184.

the plosive is released, or the *formant transitions*; and the third is how long it takes the vocal folds to start vibrating, or the *voice onset time* or *VOT*, following the release.

The center frequency of the burst in a plosive changes with the place of articulation. In English, there are three places of articulation used in plosives: bilabial, alveolar, and velar. The center frequency of the burst is low (approximately 500 Hz to 1.5 kHz) for bilabial plosives, high (above 4 kHz) for alveolar plosives, and intermediate (approximately 1.5 kHz to 4 kHz and generally just above F2 of following vowel) for velar plosives. Plosive bursts are illustrated in an idealized form in Figure 2–14.

A higher oral pressure is associated with voiceless plosives compared with their voiced counterparts, and their burst energy tends to be greater in amplitude and there is turbulence at the glottis immediately following the release, resulting in audible noise, known as *aspiration*.

The formant transition is the change in formant frequency that occurs whenever there is a change in articulation. In the case of plosives, formant transitions occur during the entry to and exit from the hold stage, and the formant frequencies change from whatever theirs were for the starting sound to whatever they are for the following sound. The formant frequencies for the plosives are defined as the effective formant frequencies during the hold stage itself, and these are known as *locus* (Latin for *place*) frequencies. Plosive formant transitions are therefore changes between the locus frequencies of the plosive and the formant frequencies of the adjacent vowel.

F1 has a locus frequency of 0 Hz for all plosives. The locus frequency for F2 varies both by plosive place of articulation as well as the associated vowel, and the locus frequency for F3 does not vary substantially. The F1 locus frequency is 0 Hz for all plosives. The F2 locus frequency for bilabial plosives is below F2 for all vowels, while for velar plosives it is above F2 for all vowels. For alveolar plosives the F2 locus frequency is around the F2 value for the vowel /E/. The F3 locus frequency for all plosives is lower than F3 for all vowels. Plosive formant transitions are illustrated in an idealized form in Figure 2–14 for the range of the

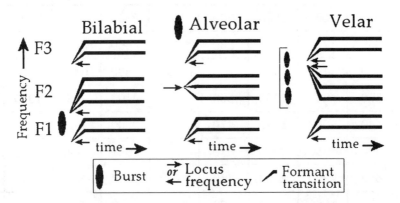

Figure 2–14. *Idealized plots of the formant transitions, formant locus frequencies, and bursts for the three places of articulation (bilabial, alveolar, velar) associated with English plosives.*

first three formant frequencies found for English vowels. It can be seen that there is a distinction available to the perceptual mechanism for identifying the place of articulation of any plosive based on the F2 locus frequency, the F2 transition, and the burst. Formant transitions in plosives last for around 10–20 ms.

Voice onset time is the time between the plosive burst, or its release, and the onset of vocal fold vibration during the following vowel. Sometimes, the VOT value can be negative when vocal fold vibration starts before the burst, when it is known as *prevoicing* or *voicing lead*. Voiceless plosives have VOT values that tend to be between approximately +25 ms to +100 ms, while voiced plosives tend to have VOT values between approximately –20 ms and +20 ms. It should be noted that these are ranges within which VOT values are typically found; no one speaker will have exact values for all utterance of a given plosive; these values will vary, for example, with speech rate. Bilabial plosives have the shortest VOT values (V+ around 5 ms, V– around 75 ms), alveolar plosives have mid values (V+ around 10 ms, V– around 85 ms), and velar plosives have the longest values (V+ around 15 ms, V– around 90 ms). In summary, the further the place of articulation is, the larger is the VOT. Variation in VOT for all English plosives can be observed in Figure 2–14.

Nasals

During the production of nasals, the velum is raised to couple in the nasal cavity and the oral cavity is blocked off. The oral cavity therefore forms a *side-branch* to the nasal cavity, which is the direct path to the outside world for sound. This side-branch is largest for the bilabial nasal /m/, shorter for the alveo-lar nasal /n/, and shortest for the velar nasal /N/. The nasal cavity has a formant structure as does any acoustic cavity, but it cannot be changed in volume, and therefore it is similar for all sounds involving the nasal cavity. The main acoustic property is the nasal formant, sometimes referred to as a *nasal murmur*, which has a frequency of around 300 Hz.

The effect of a side-branch on the overall acoustic output spectrum is that energy at its formant frequencies tends to be absorbed within the side-branch itself, thereby removing it from the sound that reaches the outside world. Removing energy in a particular formant band has the effect of creating a dip in the overall frequency response, which appears as an inverted-formant and is often called an *anti-resonance*. The nasal anti-resonances for /m/, /n/, and /N/ are located at approximately 1 kHz, 3.5 kHz, and 5 kHz, respectively (notice that, as one might expect, the frequency of the anti-resonance is higher when the cavity is smaller). Formant transitions are just as important an acoustic cue for nasals as they are for plosives, and the F2 locus frequencies are typically around 1.2 kHz for /m/, 1.8 kHz for /n/, and 2.1 kHz for /N/. The overall amplitude in nasals is considerably lower than that for vowels due to the relatively small nostril opening compared to lip opening and the presence of energy removing inverted formants or anti-resonances.

Fricatives

Fricatives result from a narrow constriction being formed in the vocal tract, through which air is passed at a velocity sufficiently high for turbulent air flow (which is the voiceless sound source that is heard as noise) to result. Fricatives last from around 50 ms up to 200 ms, which is rather longer than for other consonants; indeed, fricative duration is greater than affricates for the two fricatives concerned (/S/ and /Z/), and the affricates last longer than plosives. Fricatives can be voiced or unvoiced (see Table 2–1), and voiced fricatives have a double sound source (the vibrating vocal folds as well as air being forced through a narrow constriction), which results in the turbulence being pulsed on and off as the vocal folds open and close.

The effect of the sound modifiers during fricative production depends on the place of articulation and the volume of the acoustic cavity between it and the lips. The larger this cavity, the lower is its resonant frequency. So as the fricative place of articulation moves from dental to glottal in the order /T/ and /D/, /f/ and /v/, /s/ and /z/, /S/ and /Z/, /h/, the cavity in front of the constriction up to the lips becomes larger, and therefore the resonant frequency becomes lower. The alveolar (/s/, /z/) and palatal (/S/, /Z/) fricatives exhibit the greatest acoustic energy compared with the others. The spectral energy in alveolar fricatives lies above approximately 4 kHz, while that for palatal fricatives is above approximately 2.5 kHz. The spectral spread of energy for the labiodental (/f/, /v/) and dental fricatives (/T/, /D/) tends to be rather more diffuse because the resonant frequencies are less well defined.

Once again the F2 transition into and out of fricatives is an important acoustic cue for fricative identification, particularly in the case of the labiodental (/f/, /v/) and dental (/T/, /D/—which have the least well defined resonance frequencies), and their loci are usually found around 1 kHz and 1.4 kHz, respectively. However, the glottal fricative /h/ usu-

ally exhibits no formant transitions since it is produced at the glottis and no significant articulatory change is required for the onset of voicing. During /h/, the vocal tract is already configured for the following vowel, and the noise energy associated with /h/ usually exhibits the formant frequencies of the following vowel.

Affricates

The English affricates /tS/ and dZ/ consist of a plosive and fricative in sequence. The plosive portion has the acoustic characteristics of /t/ and /d/, respectively, but with little formant transition into the fricative since the change in articulation is small. The fricative portion is shorter than it would be if it were being produced as a stand-alone fricative. Otherwise the acoustics of affricates can be described in terms of those of the plosive and fricative of which they are comprised.

Semivowels

The four semivowels (/w/, /r/, /l/, /j/) appear structurally in English as consonants (consider their positions in words such as: *you, zoo, woo, right, light, bight, white*), and they have much in common with diphthongs in terms of their acoustic structure. However, they last for a shorter time (around 100 ms) compared to diphthongs (approximately 250 ms). The formants associated with /w/ and /j/ are very close in frequency to the vowels /u/ and /i/, respectively, since they have similar places of articulation. The main acoustic feature that characterizes /r/ is an extreme lowering of F3 (the lowest value found in English), so that it is close to F2, and this and the associated formant transitions enable the identification of /r/. During /l/, F3 is higher than for /r/ and hardly varies in the context of surrounding vowels. The position of F2 allows the semivowels to be distinguished as it is low for /u/, in a mid position for /r/ and /l/, and high for /j/, and the F3 differences between /r/ and /l/ enable their disambiguation.

Perturbation Theory

The formant properties of the vocal tract are not easy to predict directly from the tract shape. As more is understood about the acoustics of singing and speech, and as voice teachers are beginning to think and read more about voice production and explain it to their students in terms of acoustics, it can be very useful to make more direct connections between articulation and changes to the acoustic output. This can be done using *perturbation theory*, which indicates how the natural resonances of a tube (or formants of the oral cavity) will be altered

in frequency as the tube (oral cavity) is constricted or expanded (perturbed) at different positions along its length.

Figure 2–15 shows the first three acoustic pressure standing wave modes of a constant diameter tube closed at one end (recall from Chapter 1 that the necessary conditions for establishing the nature of pressure standing waves are that there is a pressure maximum at the closed end, or a pressure antinode, and no pressure variation at the open end, or a pressure node). In speech, the first vowel in *agog* (/@/) is produced with a relaxed oral cavity, and the diameter of the tube is reasonably constant. Based on the equation that relates frequency, wavelength, and the velocity of sound (see Chapter 1), the frequencies of these first three standing wave modes (the formant frequencies for /@/) can be calculated. The average vocal tract length for an adult male is 17.5 cm (or 0.175 m), and the velocity of sound in air is 344 meters per second at room temperature.

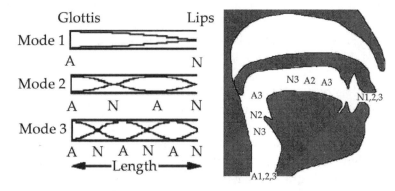

Figure 2–15. *The first three acoustic pressure standing wave modes (the first three formants) for a tube closed at one end (left) and the positions of the nodes (N) and antinodes (A) in the neutral relaxed oral cavity, which would produce the vowel /@/ (right). The necessary conditions for acoustic pressure standing wave modes are an antinode (A) at the glottis (closed) end and a node (N) at the lip (open) end.*

From the figure it can be seen that the first mode has a wavelength that is 4 times the length of the tube, so its first formant frequency ($F1_{(/@/)}$) is:

$$F1_{(/@/)} = \left(\frac{c}{4L_c}\right) = \qquad (2.2)$$

$$\left(\frac{344}{4 \times 0.175}\right) = 491 \text{ Hz}$$

Its second mode has a wavelength that is ¾ of the tube length, so its second formant frequency ($F2_{(/@/)}$) is:

$$F2_{(/@/)} = \left(\frac{3c}{4L_c}\right) = \text{ or } 3F1_{(/@/)} = \qquad (2.3)$$

$$(3 \times 491) = 1474 \text{ Hz}$$

Its third mode has a wavelength that is 1¼ of the tube length, so its third formant frequency ($F3_{(/@/)}$) is:

$$F3_{(/@/)} = \left(\frac{5c}{4L_c}\right) = \text{ or } 5F1_{(/@/)} = \qquad (2.4)$$

$$(5 \times 491) = 2457 \text{ Hz}$$

For convenience, these formant frequency values for the neutral adult male vocal tract (the vowel /@/) are generally approximated as a rule of thumb to: $F1_{(/@/)} = 500$ Hz; $F2_{(/@/)} = 1500$ Hz; $F3_{(/@/)} = 2500$ Hz.

Each mode has particular positions along the length of the tube where the acoustic pressure is either zero (node or N) or a maximum (antinode or A) as shown in the left-hand plot in Figure 2–15. The plot on the right side of the figure relates these directly to the vocal tract for the neutral vowel /@/, which is essentially a constant diameter tube. Notice that every formant has a volume pressure node at the lips and an antinode at the glottis. The other nodes and antinodes for the second and third for-

mants occur at distances appropriate to their standing wave patterns shown in the left-hand plot in the figure. Starting with the configuration for the neutral vowel /@/, the formant changes associated with other vowels can be predicted using perturbation theory.

Articulation within the oral cavity (using the tongue, jaw, or lips) has the effect of squeezing or enlarging the tube (the perturbation). The effect that this change has on any particular formant can be predicted by considering where the perturbation is with respect to its node or antinode based on the following principles:

- A constriction near a pressure node lowers that formant's frequency.
- A constriction near a pressure antinode raises that formant's frequency.
- Lengthening the vocal tract raises all formant frequencies. This can be done using lip protrusion and/or larynx lowering.
- Shortening the vocal tract lowers all formant frequencies. This can be done using lip retraction and/or larynx raising.

Figure 2–16 shows the effect of a constriction separately (for clarity) for each of the first three formants (F1, F2, F3), using a plus sign (+) to indicate that a constriction at that point would raise the formant frequency (because it is close to a pressure antinode), and a minus sign (−) to indicate that a constriction at that point would lower the formant frequency (because it is near to a pressure node). The size of the plus or minus sign indicates how great the raising or lowering would be—this simply indicates how close that constriction

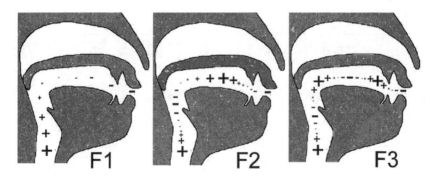

Figure 2–16. *Positive (+) and negative (–) formant frequency modification with constriction position along the oral tract for F1, F2, and F3.*

position is to the antinode or node. It is interesting to note that a lip constriction will lower the frequencies of all formants since they all have a pressure node at the lips.

For example, the vowel /i/ (front, close vowel—see Figure 2–8) has a constriction (see Figure 2–13) in the region of both A2 and A3 (see Figure 2–16), and therefore F2 and F3 are raised in frequency (see Table 2–1). The vowel /A/ has a constriction in the region of both N2 and N3, resulting in a lowering of both F2 and F3 (see Table 2–1). The vowel /u/ has lip rounding, which lowers all formant frequencies (see Table 2–1).

The relationship between the open/ close axis of the vowel quadrilateral and the first two formants can be seen inferred from Figure 2–16. The first formant is lowered as the tongue moves from open to close. The second formant is lowered as the tongue constriction moves from front to back.

Singers make a number of articulation changes as they strive to achieve their appropriate acoustic output. Perturbation theory enables the effect on formant frequencies to be predicted as a result of these variations. This is something which will become increasingly important as more interest is shown by singers and their teachers in understanding the acoustics of singing and the effect that their articulation gestures are having on their overall acoustic output.

Formants in Singing

During singing, a wide range of f0 is used, as indicated in Figure 2–10. One major consequence of this is that as the f0 is raised and the harmonics are spaced further apart, the formants become less well defined. For sopranos towards the top of their pitch range (notes above around D5 [587 Hz]—see Figure 2–10), vowels become indistinguishable. This is illustrated in idealized form in Figure 2–17 for the vowel in *fast* (/A/) sung on three different notes (G3, G4, G5).

The sound source is harmonic, and the sound modifier response is shown for /A/ with its first three formant positions indicated (review Figure 2–13 and its discussion). The output is the result of the harmonics of the sound source having their amplitudes changed by the sound modifiers (vocal tract), and this can be seen in Figures 2–13 and 2–17. For G3, the formant positions are very clear

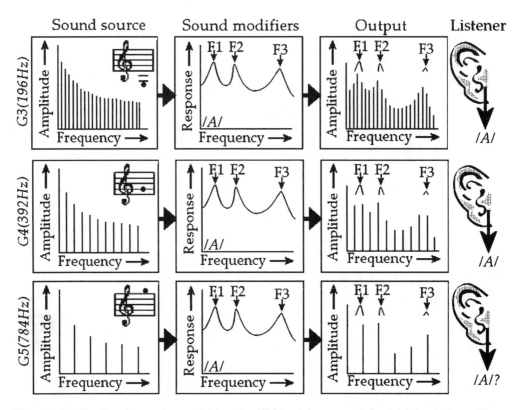

Figure 2–17. *The loss of vowel identity (/A/ in this example) at high pitches. Three pitches are illustrated (G3, G4, G5) along with their sung (voiced) sound source, sound modifier (vocal tract) response and the outputs for the vowel /A/. Formant positions are indicated, and it can be seen that the vowel identity is not clear for G5 due to the wide harmonic spacing of its sound source.*

in the output spectrum because there are plenty of harmonics populating the frequency spectrum to retain clearly the shape of the sound modifier response. This enables the listener to identify the formants and recognize the vowel as /A/. One octave higher (G4), the number of harmonics is halved (the f0 when going up one octave is doubled and therefore so is the harmonic spacing), but there are still sufficient harmonics available to retain the shape of the sound modifier response, and the three formants can be identified and the vowel identified. At G5 the number of harmonics is halved again, and now there are not enough harmonics present to retain the shape of

the sound modifier response and vowel identification becomes ambiguous.

Figure 2–17 also allows another very important principle to be reinforced. The exact frequencies of the formants are not those of the harmonics that have the peak amplitudes in an output spectrum unless there just happens to be a harmonic sitting at exactly the frequency of the formant. This is particularly clear for G4 and G5 in this example. Formant identification involves inferring the shape of the sound modifier response curve over the harmonic amplitudes.

Sopranos make particular sound modifier adjustments when singing notes above about C5 (523 Hz) where vowels start to become less distinct. They aim to position the lower formants over individual harmonics of the excitation so that they are transmitted via the vocal tract with the greatest amplitude, and thus they produce sounds of high intensity which will project well. The vocal tract is, in effect, being "tuned in" to each individual note sung, and often particular vowels are associated with each pitch as a reminder. This does not affect how the text is perceived since the harmonics are becoming so far apart that relative formant positions in frequency are lost (see Figure 2–17).

Tenors do not need to adopt such a strategy since the ratio between their formant frequencies and f0 of the higher notes in the tenor's range is higher than that for sopranos (see Table 2–2). However, there is a need to project above accompaniment, particularly when this is a full orchestra, the performance is in a large auditorium, and amplification is not being used. The acoustic result of projection is illustrated in Figure 2–18, which shows idealized spectra for a spoken version of the text, the orchestral accompaniment alone, and the orchestra accompanying the text sung by a professional singer. The plots have been amplitude normalized for comparison convenience (The singer cannot read text as loudly as an orchestra plays!).

The spectrum of the spoken text has the same general shape as that for the orchestra playing alone. When the orchestra accompanies a professional singer singing the text, the spectrum has a shape similar to both the speech and orchestral accompaniment at low frequencies, but there is an additional broad peak between approximately 2.5 kHz and 4 kHz, centered at about 3 kHz. This peak relates to the acoustic output from the singer. Its similarity to formants in the vocal tract response has been noted, and it is therefore known as the *singer's formant*, which is discussed in detail in Sundberg (1989). The singer's formant helps the singer to be heard above an accompanying orchestra because it lies in a spectral region occupied only at a low level by the orchestral output. This is the characteristic *ring*, and it results from lowering the larynx and widening the pharynx, something teachers are aiming for when suggesting, for example, that

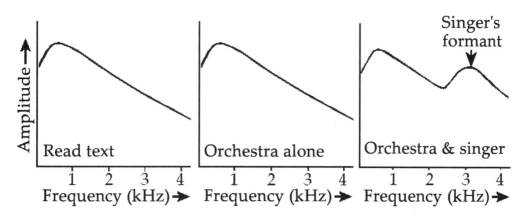

Figure 2–18. *Idealized spectra for a read text (left), the orchestral accompaniment alone (middle), and the orchestra accompanying the text sung by a professional singer (right). The peak in the accompanied singing is known as the "singer's formant."*

pupils "sing on the point of the yawn," or "sing as if they have swallowed an apple which has stuck in their throat."

DEVELOPING AND MAINTAINING A HEALTHY PROFESSIONAL VOICE

Computers in Voice Training

Modern multimedia office and home computers are more than capable of analyzing the acoustic output of speech or singing fast enough to put the result on screen with no noticeable delay, or in *real time*. Computers are now being used to support the voice training process, and a basic understanding of the acoustics of voice is important for anyone intending to interpret such displays. This section provides some examples of the kind of displays that are being used in singing training, and these are presented as a means of illustrating some of the key points in relation to the acoustics of professional voice production.

Figure 2–19 shows the speech pressure waveform and narrowband and wideband spectrograms (see Chapter 1)

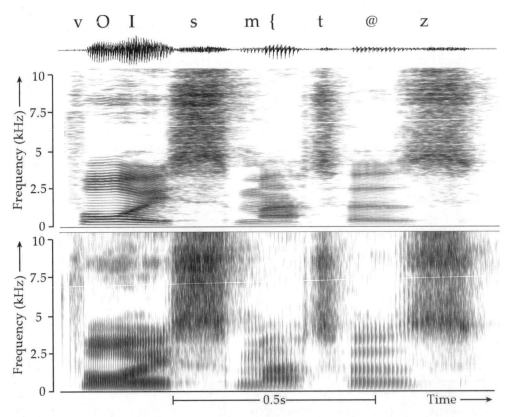

Figure 2–19. *SAMPA transcription, speech pressure waveform (upper), and narrowband (middle) and wideband (lower) spectrograms of "voice matters" spoken by an adult male.*

for "voice matters" spoken by an adult male. An approximately time-aligned SAMPA transcription is provided to help identify individual sounds.

The underlying structure in the narrowband spectrogram is horizontal due to its good frequency resolution, and during the voiced sections (the sounds /OI/, /m{/, /@z/), these horizontal lines are harmonics of f0. Since harmonics are integer multiples of f0, they are spaced equally in frequency. The underlying pitch contour is shown in the movement of the harmonics. The wideband spectrogram has good time resolution, which manifests itself during voiced speech as vertical lines, known as *striations*. Each striation represents an individual vocal fold closure. During the voiceless sounds, such as the consonant /s/ in *voice*, the acoustic excitation is noise-based and no harmonics or striations are visible in the narrow- or wideband spectrograms, respectively. Evidence of a nasal murmur (energy around 300 Hz) and an anti-resonance (lack of energy just under 1 kHz, that is) is particularly visible on the narrowband spectrogram during the nasal consonant /m/. During voiceless sounds, the representation of the noise remains essentially horizontal in the narrowband and vertical in the wideband spectrogram, respectively.

Formant frequencies would usually be measured on a wideband spectrogram since its striations cross the full extent of the formant bands themselves, whereas the harmonics on the narrowband spectrogram only indicate when they are within a formant (see Chapter 1). The first, second, and third formant transitions during the diphthong /OI/ can be clearly seen on both spectrograms. Any duration measurement would be most accurately measured from the wideband spectrogram due to its shorter time response; for example, the release of /t/ in *matters* is cleanly defined in time on the wideband spectrogram, but appears more spread out in time on the narrowband spectrogram.

Figure 2–20 shows an f0 plot and a narrowband spectrogram for the vowel /A/ sung in an "untrained" and "trained" style on an arpeggio from the first author's WinSingad singing training software. Each individual note of the arpeggio can be seen in the f0 plot, and the singer's formant region is that between the two horizontal dashed lines. It can be seen that there is energy in this region only when singing in the trained style. In addition, evidence of increased vibrato in the trained version can be seen as an undulation in the harmonics, which is essentially absent in the untrained version. Notice how the undulations are greater for the higher harmonics. This is because the variation on f0 is multiplied by the appropriate integer harmonic number and therefore appears that many times larger. For example, if the vibrato variation is ±10 Hz on f0, it will be ±20 Hz (2 × 10 Hz) on the second harmonic, ±30 Hz (3 × 10 Hz) on the third harmonic, and so on.

Figure 2–21 shows a display of oral tract area between the larynx and the lips that can be viewed in real time using the first author's WinSingad singing training software. It provides an indication of a rather more unusual display that can be achieved using a standard computer, and it gives the voice professional access to information about the shape of the oral cavity during the production of a sound. Here, the relative sizes of the lip opening as well as the

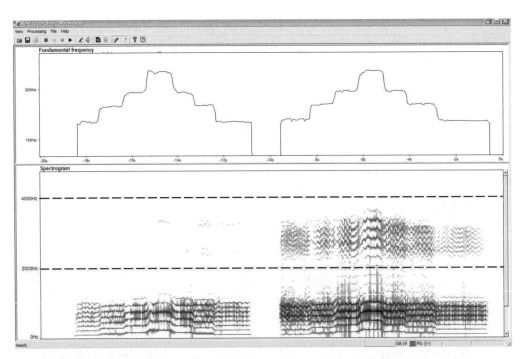

Figure 2–20. *Fundamental frequency (upper) and narrowband spectrogram (lower) from the first author's WinSingad singing training software of the vowel /A/ sung in an "untrained" (left) and "trained" (right) style on an arpeggio.*

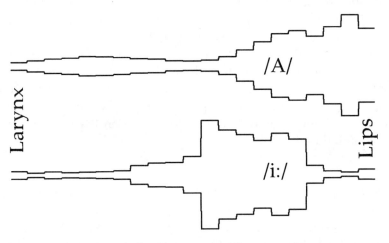

Figure 2–21. *Oral tract (mouth) area plots available in real time from the first author's WinSingad singing training software for the vowels /A/ and /i/ sung by an adult male.*

front and back cavities of the mouth during the vowels /A/ and /i/ can be directly compared. From the plot, it can be seen that in this example the sung /i/ vowel involves a back mouth area that is larger than would be typically found during a spoken version. For this /A/ vowel, there is evidence of increased opening in the left-hand half of the tube, which is the pharyngeal region above the larynx.

The singer's formant and vibrato are usually very clearly seen in spectrograms of professional opera singers. Figure 2–22 shows narrowband spectrograms for three professional tenors [Pavarotti (Pav), Carreras (Car), and Domingo (Dom)] singing the last three syllables of the second (unaccompanied) "*(vit)toria*" from Act 2 of *Tosca* by Puccini from commercial compact disk recordings. Under each is plotted a long-term average spectrum (LTAS) of the material shown in the spectrogram. The singer's formant (SF) region is indicated on the spectrograms and the LTAS plots, and it can be seen that all three tenors have a very strong energy boost in this region. In addition, all three use very significant amounts of vibrato. The LTAS plot provides another way of looking at the data, especially when comparisons are being made. It can be seen that each tenor has his own pattern of energy distribution between the singer's formant region and the rest of the spectrum. In this example, Domingo has the highest singer's formant energy relative to the lower frequencies, with a rapid reduction above 3 kHz.

These plots serve to show how individual each and every voice is, even for those at the top of the singing profession. This is one of the very special captivating features of human voice production that tantalizes those working on speech and singing analysis and synthesis. Synthetic speech is highly intelligible, but it is clearly the output from a computer; it lacks those idiosyncratic elements that convey naturalness.

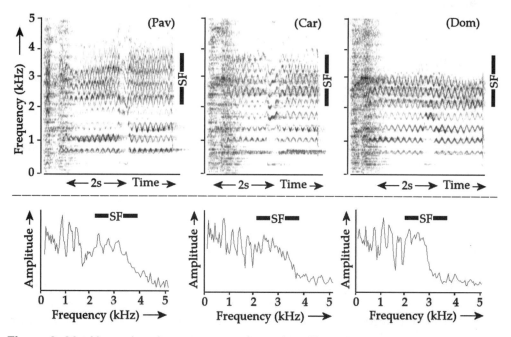

Figure 2–22. *Narrowband spectrograms (upper) and long-term average spectra (LTAS) of the whole spectrogram (lower) of commercial compact disk recordings of three professional tenors [Pavarotti (Pav), Carreras (Car), and Domingo (Dom)] singing the last three syllables of the second (unaccompanied) "(vit)toria" from Act 2 of Tosca by Puccini. The singer's formant region is indicated in each plot as "SF."*

Tips for Maintaining a Healthy Voice

Healthy voice production requires that the instrument itself is in good working order. In the same way that athletes need to prepare their bodies before a competitive event, professional voice users will do the same. Of course, not everyone will become a professional voice user, but there are a number of useful and straightforward things that everyone can do to keep his or her voice healthy. Three aspects are covered briefly by way of practical guidance here:

1. Preparing the voice and voice use
2. Drink and food for the healthy voice
3. Environmental considerations

Vocal Warm-Up and Cool-Down

Healthy voice function requires that the muscles in the neck area, which include those that support the larynx, are relaxed, so that the necessary muscular gestures needed for voice production can operate over their full range of movement. Tension in the neck muscles is one result of the everyday stress of 21st century life; it often manifests itself with raised shoulders, and a shortened neck with the head pulled down towards the ribcage. Such a position is completely inappropriate for healthy voice production, since the space within which the larynx is located is severely restricted, the vocal tract space immediately above the larynx is reduced, and the muscles that control larynx function have little or no room for maneuver.

Preparing the voice should be thought through in terms of warming up and cooling down each of the three parts of the vocal instrument: the *power source*, the *sound source* for voiced sounds, and the *sound modifiers*, or the breathing system, the larynx, and the moving parts of the vocal tract. Warming up should be part of preparing for a speaking or singing engagement, and afterwards the voice should be cooled down to return to a rested state. The same exercises can be used for warming up and cooling down.

Warming up or cooling down the breathing system involves setting and maintaining an appropriate posture and using abdominal and lower rib cage breathing as described in Voice Production. It is very important to stand tall and straight, and there are many ways of gaining good posture, for example, by taking voice training lessons and/or sessions in Alexander or Feldenkrais technique, pilates, or yoga. Breathing can be self-monitored in front of a mirror to check that the chest and shoulders remain still, by placing hands on the lowest ribs to check for *bellows* movement, and by placing a hand over the navel to check for abdominal breathing (see Figure 2–2). Sustaining long /f/, /s/, or /S/ sounds (see Table 2–1) when breathing out serves to exercise and warm up the muscles associated with breathing out.

The sound source for voiced sounds should be warmed up gently, and many singers use a technique known as *sirening*. This involves making the final sound of the word *sing*, or /N/ (see Table 2–1), and gliding over a wide pitch range a few times. The idea is to push the extremes further up and down in pitch each time if possible, while being careful not to strain the voice.

Warming up or cooling down those parts of the vocal tract that move involves exercising each in turn. The main elements are the lips, tongue, and jaw. A lip trill is a good exercise, which involves making the lips vibrate together like a braying horse, and repeating this on three to five out-breaths. The tongue can be warmed up by sticking it out and lapping (flicking the tongue tip in and out of the mouth, contacting the upper lip each time) like a cat when drinking water or milk. This should be sustained for, say, 15 to 20 seconds. The jaw should be opened to its extreme, than moved in a rectangle from bottom left to bottom right to top right to top left 5 or 10 times.

These suggestions are offered to provide a starting point. Professional voice users and their teachers tend to develop their own exercises, and there are many potential variants. The important thing about voice exercises is to make the moving parts move over their full range in a gentle manner at first when warming up and finally when cooling down. It should be remembered, though, that there is no substitute for seeking advice from a voice teacher who can make observations and provide proper feedback specific to the student's needs. Even just a few lessons can offer significant benefits, especially in the early stages.

In terms of voice use, treat the voice with respect and avoid overuse whenever possible. Shouting and speaking loudly are best avoided if possible. Enunciating words more clearly by exaggerating consonants and vowels and speaking more slowly enable the loudness level to be reduced, and it encourages the listener to listen more intently, thereby paying more attention to what is being said. Throat clearing by coughing involves closing the glottis, building up lung air pressure from below, and then opening the glottis rapidly, releasing a very rapid flow of air. This puts additional strain on the vocal folds and it is best avoided if possible.

Swallowing can help, and speaking through the cough without "giving in" to it is what many public speakers strive to achieve.

Drink and Food for the Healthy Voice

Like any instrument, a little care and attention paid to the routine operation of the voice production mechanism helps to ensure trouble-free working. Recalling that the vocal folds close and open very many times during speech (over 1 million times per day estimated for a teacher, as stated in the section Voice Production) or singing (over 150,000 times in 5 minutes estimated for an operatic soprano, as stated in Voice Production), attention should be paid to keeping the vocal folds properly and regularly lubricated. This is essential in helping to avoid voice problems such as vocal fold nodules or polyps. Water is the best lubricant, and one can never drink too much of it. Professional actors and singers reckon that around four liters per day is required to keep their voices in good order, and they are rarely seen in rehearsals without a water bottle. As a practical goal for everyday voice use, a target of one and a half to two liters per day is suggested as being perhaps more appropriate.

The larynx itself does not require such copious amount of water; other organs such as the kidneys and liver need to be sufficiently supplied with water before there is surplus to supply the vocal system adequately for healthy and prolonged voice use. Starting every day by drinking about three quarters of a liter of water before saying anything to anyone helps prepare the voice for the day ahead. There are two useful indicators as to whether one has drunk sufficient water for maintaining a healthy voice: (a) there should be plenty of saliva in the mouth, which should not feel at all dry, and (b) urine should be a pale color and not particularly yellow, or *pee pale*.

Other drinks are generally not so good for the voice if they contain substances that tend to have a drying effect, such as caffeine or alcohol. Sugary drinks are not good because the sugar content tends to make saliva more viscous. Products that contain nonsoluble fats are not good because they tend to inhibit proper lubrication, and they cannot be cleared from the vocal tract with saliva or water (this is readily confirmed by sucking on a piece of chocolate or eating a banana and sensing how the mouth feels afterwards). It is, though, possible to clear these fats from the vocal tract by adding an acid to break them down into soluble fats. The most effective acid is lemon juice, and a few drops in water works well. Grapefruit juice is also good, and orange juice does have a useful effect. Many who use their voices regularly carry lemon juice around in the form of either a squeezy lemon (as is often used for cooking) or *pure lemon juice* in a bottle.

By way of a summary, Table 2–3 lists drinks that are good for the voice and those that should be avoided for 1 to 2 hours before a speaking or singing engagement. One drink (red port) is listed as being good as a vocal *first aid*, and many professional voice users are aware of its usefulness when the voice is somewhat sore and tired. The alcohol helps soothe the throat, and it contains chemicals that appear to aid lubrication and fat breakdown. It should be noted that it is only the first shot that helps, and that it is only *red* port, and not tawny or white port, that works.

In terms of foods, the guiding principle is to avoid fatty foods in the period 1 to 2 hours before speaking or singing for prolonged periods, and to eat fruit. Unfortunately, bananas, which are an excellent source of sustenance, are for most people an exception to this, because they have a significant fat content. Table 2–3 lists foods that are good and those that should be avoided before singing or speaking.

It is important to note that the drinks and foods listed in Table 2–3 as being best avoided only apply to the period *1 to 2 hours before a significant speaking or singing engagement*. Outside this time, normal dietary habits can, of course, be followed. However, large late night meals should be avoided since sleeping with a bloated stomach can encourage gastric reflux (stomach acids escaping into the throat region), which tends to irritate the laryngeal region and can be harmful to the voice. If anything like this is of concern, seek professional medical help.

Environmental Considerations

The local environment can have a significant effect on vocal health, particularly in terms of keeping the system moist to maintain appropriate lubrication. A dry throat is often experienced when the local environment has low humidity, and it is important to be aware of this and to drink extra water. Humidity is particularly low in aircraft and in surroundings that are air conditioned, but usually water is readily available.

When there is considerable competing acoustic noise locally, for example, in aircraft, some trains, other forms of transport, building sites, school classrooms, swimming pools, and sports halls, there is a natural tendency to compensate by speaking more loudly or shouting. This happens automatically, and if it continues for any length of time, vocal

Table 2–3. Drinks and foods that are good and best avoided before speaking or singing for prolonged periods. Note that drinks and foods listed as being best avoided are only for the period 1 to 2 hours before a significant speaking or singing engagement; outside this time, normal dietary habits can be followed.

DRINKS	
Good	**Best avoided (1–2 hours beforehand)**
water	coffee
herbal tea	caffeinated tea
acidic fruit juice (e.g., lemon, orange, grapefruit)	alcoholic drinks
	sugary drinks
one shot of red port (once only as first aid)	fizzy drinks
	milk
	milkshakes

FOODS	
Good	**Best avoided (1–2 hours beforehand)**
fruit (e.g., apples, oranges, strawberries, grapes, tomatoes)	chocolate
	cheese
	yogurt
	cream
	ice cream
	cake
	cookies
	bananas

fatigue could well result. By becoming more aware of such spaces through more focused conscious listening, it is possible to know when to reduce voice usage by saying less, and to make oneself understood by enunciating words more clearly to allow speech to remain at a lower loudness level.

Smoky environments can cause irritation and dryness and are best avoided whenever possible. The presence of noxious fumes can also cause throat clearing, which should be reduced to a minimum.

Maintaining a Healthy Voice— Summary

Maintaining a healthy voice is important for everyone who uses her voice for whatever purpose, even when there is no specific vocal load in addition to everyday living. Given its importance, a summary of the main tips is presented below to serve as an *aide memoire*. It is very worthwhile to adopt one or more of these tips into the regular routine.

- Use some form of vocal warm-up before long periods of voice use
- Drink plenty of water regularly
- Avoid smoky environments
- Avoid noxious fumes
- Avoid shouting
- Avoid heavy meals late at night
- Before a major speaking or singing event:
  - Choose foods carefully during preceding 1 to 2 hours
  - Choose drinks carefully during preceding 1 to 2 hours
  - Rest the voice
  - Refrain from heavy throat clearing
  - Keep conversations short
  - Drink plenty of water when flying or in air-conditioned spaces
- Use some form of vocal cool-down after long periods of voice use

Remember, you only have one voice and its laryngeal working parts are small, vulnerable, and delicate. Vocal communication is so fundamental to our everyday as well as our professional lives— look after it properly.

convenient organization for the acoustic descriptions of these sounds. Knowledge of the acoustics of speech and singing can aid understanding for both voice teacher and voice student as they work together to build a vocal sound. Today's multimedia PCs enable acoustic analyses to be carried out so that the waveform and spectral features described can be readily observed. Indeed, there are now software packages available (look under Further Reading for some Web links) that enable these displays to be provided immediately, thereby providing real-time visual feedback of the acoustic patterns. Today's voice students are demanding explanations that incorporate both physiological and acoustic descriptions; this chapter sets out to provide the latter.

For the performer there are a number of practical issues that are important for vocal health and these have been described. In particular, if life changes are made to take account of the issues to do with food and drink as well as the environment, a performer stands to make significant gains in vocal agility, control of the vocal instrument, and performance confidence.

Communicating with others is as much about how the message is said or sung as it is about the content of the message itself. Treat your voice properly and it will serve you well.

SUMMARY

The human vocal instrument can produce a wide variety of sounds, the majority of which are used for communication. The sounds of English have been explored in terms of their phonetic labels of voice, place, and manner, thereby providing a

FURTHER READING

Voice Production

Ashby, M., & Maidment, J. (2006). *Introducing phonetic science*. Cambridge, UK: Cambridge University Press.

Bunch, M. (1997). *The dynamics of the singing voice.* Vienna: Springer-Verlag.

Catford, J. C. (1977). *Fundamental problems in phonetics.* Edinburgh, UK: Edinburgh University Press.

Chapman, J. (2006). *Singing and teaching singing: A holistic approach to classical voice.* San Diego, CA: Plural.

Harris, T., Harris, S., Rubin, J. S., & Howard, D. M. (1998). *The voice clinic handbook.* London: Whurr.

Ladefoged, P. (1975). *A course in phonetics.* New York: Harcourt Brace Jovanovich.

Proctor, D. F. (1980). *Breathing, speech and song.* Vienna: Springer-Verlag.

Smith, B., & Sataloff, R. T. (2000). *Choral pedagogy.* San Diego, CA: Singular.

Titze, I. (1994). *Principles of voice production* Upper Saddle River, NJ: Prentice Hall.

Van den Berg, J. W. (1958). Myoelastic-aerodynamic theory of voice production. *Journal of Speech and Hearing Research, 1,* 227–244.

Wells, J. C. (1989). Computer coded phonemic notation of individual languages of the European Community [SAMPA transcription]. *Journal of the International Phonetic Association, 19,* 32–54.

Borden, G. J., & Harris, K. S. (1980). *Speech science primer.* Baltimore: Williams & Wilkins.

Dejonckere, P. H., Hirano, M., & Sundberg, J. (1995). *Vibrato.* San Diego, CA: Singular.

Fry, D. B. (1979). *The physics of speech.* Cambridge, UK: Cambridge University Press.

Howard, D. M. (1995). Variation of electrolaryngographically derived closed quotient for trained and untrained adult singers. *Journal of Voice, 9*(2), 163–172.

Howard, D. M., & Angus, J. A. S. (2006). *Acoustics and psychoacoustics* (3rd ed.). Oxford, UK: Focal Press.

Howard, D. M., Lindsey, G. A., & Allen, B. (1990). Towards the quantification of vocal efficiency. *Journal of Voice, 4*(3), 205–212. [See also errata (1991). *Journal of Voice, 5*(1), 93–95.

Kent, R. D., & Read, C. (1992). *The acoustic analysis of speech.* San Diego, CA: Singular.

Rothenberg, M. (1992). A multi-channel electroglottograph. *Journal of Voice, 6*(1), 36–43.

Sundberg, J. (1974). Articulatory interpretation of the "singing formant." *Journal of the Acoustical Society of America, 55,* 838–844.

Sundberg, J. (1987). *The science of the singing voice.* Dekalb: Northern Illinois University Press.

Acoustics of the Vocal Output

Abberton, E. R. M., Howard, D. M., & Fourcin, A. J. (1989). Laryngographic assessment of normal voice: A tutorial. *Clinical Linguistics and Phonetics, 3*(3), 281–296.

Ashby, M., & Maidment, J. (2006). *Introducing phonetic science.* Cambridge, UK: Cambridge University Press.

Baken, R. J. (1987). *Clinical measurement of speech and voice.* London: Taylor and Francis.

Baken, R. J., & Danilof, R. G. (1991). *Readings in clinical spectrography of speech.* San Diego, CA: Singular.

Barlow, C. A., & Howard, D. M. (2005). Electrolaryngographically derived voice source changes of child and adolescent singers. *Logopedics Phoniatrics Vocology, 30*(3/4), 147–157.

Developing and Maintaining a Healthy Professional Voice

Howard, D. M., Welch, G. F., Brereton, J., Himonides, E., DeCosta, M., Williams, J., et al. (2004). WinSingad: A real-time display for the singing studio. *Logopedics Phoniatrics Vocology, 29*(3), 135–144.

Howard, D. M., Welch, G. F., Brereton, J., Himonides, E., DeCosta, M., Williams, J., et al. (2005). Are real-time displays of benefit in the singing studio? An exploratory study. *Journal of Voice, 21*(1), 20–34.

Nair, G. (1999). *Voice tradition and technology: A state-of-the-art studio.* San Diego, CA: Singular.

Rossiter, D., Howard, D. M., & DeCosta, M. (1996). Voice development under training with and without the influence of real-time visually presented feedback. *Journal of the Acoustical Society of America, 99*(5), 3253–3256.

Rossiter, D. P., Howard, D. M., & Downes, M. (1995). A real-time LPC-based vocal tract area display for voice development. *Journal of Voice, 8*(4), 314–319.

Sataloff, R. T. (1998). *Vocal health and pedagogy*. San Diego, CA: Singular.

Smith, B., & Sataloff, R. T. (2000). *Choral pedagogy*. San Diego, CA: Singular.

Thorpe, C. W., Callaghan, J., & Doorn, J. V. (1999). Visual feedback of acoustic voice features for the teaching of singing. *Australian Voice, 5,* 32–39.

Web Links to Acoustic Analysis Software Packages

Praat—http://www.praatlanguagelab.com

sfs—

WinSingad—http://winsingad.org

Singandsee—http://www.singandsee.com/index.html

Vocevista—http://www.vocevista.com/

CHAPTER 3

The Voice on Location

Whenever we speak or sing, we are communicating a message to one or more listeners. Speech communication is unique to human beings, and our speech and hearing systems have evolved to enable information to be transmitted from speaker to listener acoustically over reasonable distances almost anywhere on the planet. With the desire to perform either professionally or as part of one's job as a speaker or singer in large spaces to an audience or congregation, the local environment itself (whether a concert hall, theater, opera house, lecture hall, classroom, church, cathedral, meeting room, city hall, town hall, courtroom, parliament, legislature, market, music venue, pub, nightclub, jazz club, sports hall, swimming pool, stadium, railway station, or airport) can significantly alter the acoustic pressure wave on its journey from speaker or singer to the ears of the listener(s). Even in one-to-one conversational situations in small spaces, there can be significant issues relating to the effect of the local space on the acoustic wave from the speaker. In addition, any acoustic input from elsewhere is an unwanted and therefore competing acoustic source, which can be distracting and make communication even more difficult.

Those who use their voices in their everyday professional lives, such as teachers, lawyers, actors, singers, stock market traders, clergy, lecturers, market traders, interviewers, announcers, politicians, town criers (The first author's home city, York, UK, has one!), nurses, or doctors, are competing acoustically when communicating their messages both with the local environment and any competing acoustic noise. Quite often, they will tend naturally to increase their own acoustic output to compensate by raising their own vocal effort. This has the potential to give rise to some form of vocal impairment, particularly if the speaker has had no basic training in healthy voice use. It is salutary to note that few of those engaged in these professions are offered any vocal training as part of their professional development. While the speaker is expending additional effort in the communication process itself, there is probably less attention being paid to the process of communicating fully the ideas contained in the message itself.

The local environment itself can have a very significant effect on the transmission of the acoustic pressure wave from speaker to listener. At best it can enhance the sound of the voice and make speaking easier for the speaker and understanding clearer for the listener(s). At worst it can have a detrimental effect on the sound of the voice, making speaking a struggle for the speaker and obscuring portions of the message for the listener.

This chapter explores the acoustics of enclosed spaces and discusses how it can affect the acoustics of speech production and speech perception, in terms of what positive and negative effects the local acoustic can have on speech and singing production and perception. Practical hints and tips for making the best acoustic use of the available space are provided along with suggestions as to how vocal performers can make the local acoustic work to their advantage. It also suggests modifications that might be made to the acoustics of a space to the advantage of both healthy voice production and more effortless message perception.

ACOUSTICS OF SPACES

Introduction

The acoustic elements of voice production are described in Chapter 2 in terms of the *sound source* and *sound modifiers*, where the sound source for voiced speech or sung notes is the vibrating vocal folds, and this sound is altered by the sound modifiers as it passes through the vocal tract to produce the *sound output* from the lips and/or nostrils. This model also provides the framework within which the acoustics of spaces can be usefully discussed, reviewed, and understood. The output from the speaker or singer is the *sound source* into the room, but this sound is not what is heard by the listeners since it is modified by the acoustics of the local environment before it reaches their ears. The local environment is therefore acting as a *sound modifier*, and it is the *sound output* of the local environment that is the *sound input* to each ear of each listener.

The sound modification effect of the local environment depends on the positions of the speaker or singer (the *sound source*) and the ears of the listener or the microphone (the *receiver*). It is therefore important to note that when considering the acoustics of an environment in detail, the result will be different for each sound source/listener combination. Figure 3–1 illustrates this for a speaker or singer (shown using the model provided in Figure 2–1) in an enclosed environment where there are a number of listeners. The acoustic output from the speaker or singer is the *sound source* to the environment, and the input to each ear of a listener is its *sound output* (three ears are shown in the figure). For acoustic purposes, all speech or singing is produced in a local environment, even when it is being produced outside or in an anechoic room (a room designed to produce no reflections from its walls, floor, or ceiling—*anechoic* means *no echo*) since there is always the possibility of an acoustic reflection from some object to consider. Each ear of each listener is itself a separate sound output from the room as indicated in Figure 3–1. While the differences between what each ear of

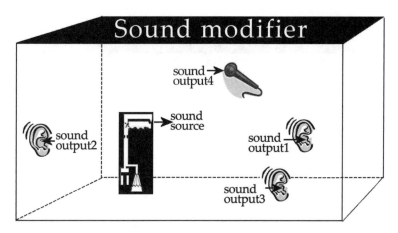

Figure 3–1. *Descriptive model as a basis for describing the effect on a vocal performance of room acoustics in terms of sound source (speaker or singer—depicted as in Figure 2–1), sound modifier (room), and sound output (sound outputs 1–3 to an ear of a listener and sound output 4 to a microphone). Note that the sound picked up by each ear of each listener is different by virtue of that listener's position in the room.*

each listener hears might be small, in some circumstances they can be important. For example, due to their relative positions within a concert hall, certain seats may provide a better listening experience than others for exactly the same source of sound.

The remainder of this section is split into three sections with respect to voice production in a space (see Figure 3–1): *sound source into a space, sound modification by a space*, and the *sound output from a space*.

Sound Source into a Space

During a vocal performance in a space, the sound that the audience is interested in is the sound input to the space by the performer(s): the *wanted sound*. The situation shown in Figure 3–1 illustrates the ideal situation where the only sound is that from the performer. No account is

being taken of other competing acoustic sounds into the space, or *unwanted sound*. No acoustic environment is completely quiet and there will always be unwanted sound, which can come from either outside the space, or within the space.

Bearing this in mind, Figure 3–2 provides an illustration of the full situation to consider with respect to the acoustics of a space, including the contributions from the wanted sound source (illustrated by the speaker model in the figure) and unwanted sounds (U). Unwanted sound from outside the space might, for example, be due to wind, thunder, rain, traffic, sirens, aircraft, or machinery. It might be noise emanating from within the building itself but outside the local environment, such as lift motors, forced air ventilation fans, air conditioning fans, water moving in the plumbing, carts being pushed down corridors, radios, recorded music, drilling, hammering, scraping, people calling to each

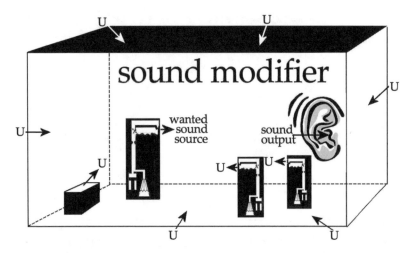

Figure 3–2. *Wanted and unwanted sound sources in a room. Unwanted sound sources (U) can be from inside or outside the room as indicated. The room acts as a sound modifier as these sounds travel to become the room's sound output into each ear of each listener.*

other, people singing, or noise from other activities in adjoining rooms.

Unwanted sound from within the space might, for example, be from others talking or making other sounds (two are illustrated in the figure), coughing, people moving around or messing about, fan noise from an overhead or computer projector, ticking or other sounds from the heating or cooling system within the room, or the clinking of glassware or other drinking vessels.

Whatever its origin and wherever we are, unwanted sound is always with us. Our world is a noisy place. In order that the message can be fully understood by each and every listener, the main acoustic changes that distinguish the sounds of the language (see Chapter 2) need to be preserved on their path to the ears of each member of the audience without additional competing noises having an adverse effect. In order to maintain the intelligibility of the spoken

or sung message, the key acoustic cues that signal each sound (see Chapter 2) and their relative timings must be preserved.

The sound source from a human vocal tract is not the same in all directions. Consider the difference in what you hear when a speaker is facing towards you or away from you in the absence of room reflections—perhaps outside on a calm day in a field. Speech sounds duller, and sounds such as /s/ and /S/ are not as loud when the speaker is facing away from you.

Sound emerges from the lips and/or nostrils of the speaker, and this sound will radiate in all directions into the space. However, the head itself acts to shadow the sound in the sound's ability to radiate behind the speaker. This effect starts to become apparent for frequencies whose wavelengths are smaller than the diameter of the head. Taking the diameter of the human head as approximately 17 cm, the frequency at which shadowing starts to occur can be calculated using equation 1.7, as follows, remembering to enter the wavelength (λ) in meters as 0.17 m.

$$f = \frac{C}{\lambda} = \frac{344}{0.17} = 2024 \text{ Hz} = \qquad (3\text{-}1)$$

2.024 kHz

This shadowing effect occurs then for frequencies above approximately 2 kHz. Conversely, for frequency components lower than 2 kHz (where λ is greater than the diameter of the head), the sound becomes less directional because the head shadowing effect has less effect. Low frequency sounds are therefore not directional and are heard at equal loudness in all directions from the speaker. Supposing a speaker started facing a listener and turned around to face away from the listener while speaking; the speech would become duller as the level of the higher frequencies reduces as the speaker turns away.

This effect is summarized in Figure 3–3, which shows that for low (around 200 Hz), mid (around 2 kHz), and high (around 5 kHz) frequencies, the voice becomes increasingly forwardly directional. In terms of level, the acoustic intensity is approximately 10 dB lower for the high frequency components compared to the low frequency components at the back compared with the front. Therefore, over the range of the first three formants (from 270 Hz to 3700 Hz —see Table 2–2), the intensity of F3 compared with F2 or F1 is highest when the listener or microphone is in front of the speaker, and progressively lower for positions further round towards behind the speaker. Notice that the mid-frequency range is radiated most efficiently about 30 degrees upwards from the mouth of the speaker, something which can be useful when placing microphones (see Chapter 5, Studio Vocal Recording).

This is part of the reason why speakers and singers are nearly always surprised

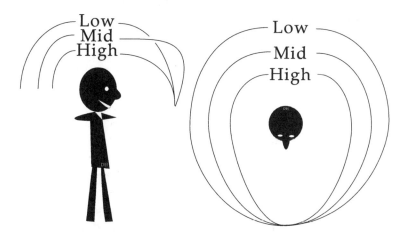

Figure 3–3. *Sketch of acoustic energy levels around the speaker/singer in the vertical (left) and horizontal (right) planes in terms of low (around 200 Hz), mid (around 2 kHz), and high (around 5 kHz) frequencies.*

by the sound of their own voices on a recording, which they sometimes find hard to believe. Our ears are behind our mouths and nostrils, and we hear our own voices as being high frequency, or *treble*, light (or low frequency, or *bass*, heavy). There is an additional factor at work; the sound of the vibrating vocal folds is also transmitted to both inner ears via bone, a phenomenon known as *bone conduction*. Bone conduction is more efficient for low frequencies and the result is that it too presents the ears with a sound that is high frequency light. In a room, the difference between listening in front of or behind the speaker becomes important when considering reflections from the wall behind the speaker or singer. The contribution that these reflections make to the total sound in the space will be high frequency light, and this should be borne in mind.

Sound Modification by a Space

An ideal sound source (one whose largest dimension is smaller than the wavelength of the highest frequency of interest to prevent sound shadowing) radiates outwards through air in all directions at the velocity of sound (344 meters per second at 20° centigrade). The acoustic energy spreads out over a spherical surface (radiation outwards in all directions at a constant velocity). As this sphere grows, the acoustic energy is spread over a larger surface area and is therefore spread more thinly. The sound intensity (energy per square meter) will be reduced, since it relates directly to how thinly the acoustic energy is spread over the surface of the sphere. The sound will be louder (higher acoustic intensity) for listeners who are closer to

the speaker. The surface area of a sphere is given by:

$$A_{sphere} = 4\pi r^2 \qquad (3\text{-}2)$$

where: A_{sphere} = the surface area of a sphere

r = the radius of the sphere (distance from sound source to listener/microphone)

If the distance between the sound source and listener (or microphone) is doubled, the surface area of the sphere increases by four (2^2), and the acoustic energy has therefore been spread out to four times its previous area, reducing it and therefore the sound intensity to a quarter of what it was before. This effect is called the *inverse square law*. For example, the sound intensity for a listener who is six meters from a sound source will be a quarter of that available to a listener who is three meters from the sound source. The inverse square law governs sound transmission in all situations. In a room, sound is reflected from and partially absorbed by the boundaries (walls, floor, and ceiling) as well as off objects in the room (tables, chairs, bookcases, furniture, people, etc.). The sound output from a room (the sound arriving at each ear of a listener—see Figure 3–2) consists of the original sound plus many versions of itself that have been reflected once or more from surfaces within the space (walls, floor, ceiling, and objects within the space).

Imagine a sound source consisting of a short, loud pulse of sound, such as a handclap. The first sound the listener hears (or a microphone picks up) will be the handclap itself after the delay needed for it to travel from the sound source's position to the listener's ear (or the microphone). This delay can be found by dividing the distance between the sound source and the ear of the listener (in meters) by the velocity of sound (344 meters per second. This first sound that the listener hears is called the *direct sound*, since it takes the direct (straight line) path to the listener (or microphone).

The next sound to reach the listener is the next shortest path, which will involve typically one reflection from the surface of an object or a room boundary. There follow a number of discrete versions of the sound that have been reflected off one or more surfaces, objects, and/or room boundaries. These are all called the *early sound*, and they are characterized by being separated in time and direction. Following the early sound, there continue to be reflections from the surfaces within the room, which arrive at each ear of the listener (or the microphone) much more closely together in time. This is because the sound can travel via such a huge number of single and multiple reflection paths that the arrival times are closely clustered. This large cluster of sounds is called the *reverberant sound*.

The direct, early, and reverberant sounds in response to a handclap are illustrated in Figure 3–4. The upper part of the figure illustrates the direct sound

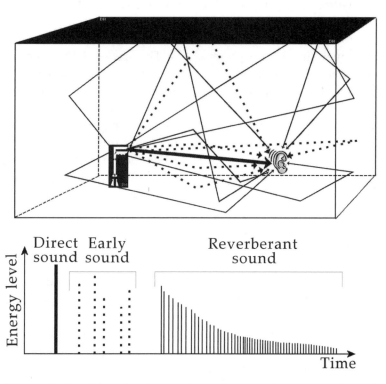

Figure 3–4. *The direct sound, early sound, and reverberant sound in a room arriving at one ear of a listener (or a microphone) illustrated as room boundary reflections (upper) and arrival times (lower).*

as well as the buildup of the early and reverberant sounds in terms of reflections from the room boundaries. The lower part of the figure shows the times of arrival at the listener of the individually reflected handclaps, and the discrete nature of the elements of the early sound can be seen as well as the close clustering of the reflections that make up the reverberant sound.

The energy levels (or *amplitudes*) of the elements of the reverberant sound die away fairly smoothly, as illustrated in Figure 3–4, in a manner that is *exponential*. This is because each element has been reflected a number of times from different surfaces around the room, so that on average, the sound energy absorbed during the transit of each element is the same over a given time. This could be thought of as a *half life* for the sound energy; the energy always decays by half over a given time. An exponential curve plots a half life decay, which is why the reverberant sound has an exponential amplitude change, or *exponential decay*. The exponential decay of the reverberant sound varies with the size of the room. For a small room the time between reflections is shorter, while for a large room the time between reflections is longer, since there is less and more time to travel, respectively. The later the arrival of a sound, the lower in level it will be due to both the inverse square law and some sound energy being absorbed at each reflection. The time taken for the sound intensity to be reduced by 60 dB after the input from the sound source has ceased is known as the *reverberation time*, which is often written as RT_{60}. A small furnished family living room might have a reverberation time of around a quarter of a second (or 250 ms),

whereas a very large space such as a cathedral might have a reverberation time of up to 10 seconds.

The discussion so far has been based on the sound input being a handclap or acoustic impulse. In the real world when someone is speaking or singing, the sound input produced into the room is essentially a continuous input. During a continuous sound input, the reverberant sound will continue to build up into a *reverberant field*. The reverberant field has three phases: the *sound buildup*, the *sound in a steady state*, and the *sound decay*, which are illustrated in Figure 3–5 for a sound input that is assumed to be constant with start and stop times as shown. The nature of the reverberant field has a direct effect on the ease with which a vocal performer can be understood and the overall vocal effort required for a successful performance.

The size of the room directly affects the buildup time, which is more rapid for a small room because the time between arrivals of the reflected elements of the sound output is shorter, and therefore the output sound level builds more rapidly. The steady state is an equilibrium position that is reached when the new sound energy input to the space is equal to the sound energy being absorbed in the space due to surface reflections and the inverse square law. Therefore the steady state level will be higher in rooms with low levels of sound absorption. When the input sound stops (see Figure 3–5), the sound energy dies away as it is absorbed by surface reflections. The decay time will therefore vary with the degree of sound absorption within a space, and it will be more rapid for spaces with high levels of sound absorption.

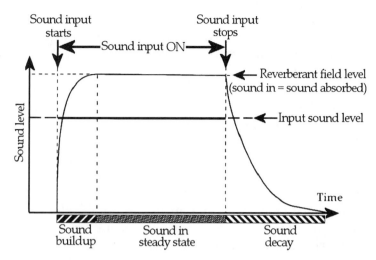

Figure 3–5. *The buildup of the reverberant field during a sound at a reasonably constant energy level. (From "Acoustics and Psychoacoustics", 3rd ed., by D. M. Howard and J. A. S. Angus, 2006, Oxford: Focal Press.*

Sound Output from a Space

The sound output from a space is the sound arriving at each ear of each listener or at a microphone (see Figure 3–1). The sound modification effect of a space adds early and reverberant sound to the direct sound as illustrated in Figure 3–4. The figure shows how the sound output consists of many copies of the original sound with different delays and amplitudes. Some of these make up the early sound and some the reverberant sound, depending on how closely together in time they arrive at each ear of each listener (or microphone). In terms of the sound output from the space, the early and reverberant sounds each have a different effect on the intelligibility and overall loudness, and it is therefore useful to consider each separately.

The nature of the early sound is specific to the positions of both the sound source and the listener or microphone as illustrated in Figure 3–4. The amplitudes of each reflection that makes up the early sound will be different, and sometimes those reflections that arrive later can have higher amplitudes than those arriving earlier, as shown in the figure. This is be because the energy lost in a particular reflection depends on the sound absorbing characteristics associated with the particular surface at which that reflection has taken place. The reflections that make up the early sound usually involve just one reflection, and they relate directly to the specific geometry of the reflecting surfaces relative to the exact positions of the sound source and listener (or microphone). The early sound therefore provides the listener with information about both the overall size of the room as well as the position of the sound source within it. Sometimes, particularly strong (high amplitude) reflections that form part of the early sound can interfere with the direct sound and make it difficult for the listener to understand the message. For this reason, control of the early sound can be very helpful, either by finding a good position for the sound source or by careful placement of acoustic reflectors close to the sound source to spread the reflections out in a diffuse fashion.

The reverberant sound is different from the early sound in that it remains constant at any listener (or microphone) position in the space. It does not vary for different sound source and/or listener positions. The reverberant sound consists of a very large number of delayed amplitude reduced versions of the sound source that arrive from all directions, and on average, these decay in an exponential fashion as illustrated in Figure 3–4. Since there are so many reflections involved, the reverberant sound will be the same at any position within the space. It is not dependent on the positions of either the sound source or the listener (or microphone). The level of the reverberant field (see Figure 3–5) will therefore also be the same at any position in the space. A space, then, is characterized by its reverberant sound, which gives it an acoustic *signature.*

This acoustic signature provides the listener with a sense of familiarity with the sound of a space. It is worth spending a moment thinking about spaces whose sound signature you are aware of, such as a bathroom, bedroom, cathedral, concert hall, swimming pool, theater, or classroom; it is their reverberant sound that provides this. Some types of music are best suited to certain spaces because of the reverberation time. A bathroom is more acoustically live than a bedroom, and many people like to sing to themselves in the bathroom but not in the bedroom as a result. Fast contrapun-

tal music is best suited to spaces with short reverberation times so that their detail is not lost. One of the most common effects used in the studio after a master recording has been made, or in *post processing*, is reverberation, in order to control the overall acoustic signature that is imparted on the resulting sound by suggesting aurally the nature of the space involved. Capturing a suitable reverberant sound is also one of the main factors that influence the placement of the microphones when making an acoustic recording within a space, and if this is done well, the addition of reverberation in the studio is not required.

One of the key issues relating to speaking or singing in public is the intelligibility of the text for the listeners. A high level of intelligibility demands that a high level of the direct sound compared to the reverberant sound reaches the ears of the listeners (or microphone). However, the level of the direct sound changes depending on the distance between the sound source and listener (or microphone) due to the inverse square law, but as described above, the level of the reverberant sound remains essentially constant anywhere in a space. Therefore the *relative* level of the direct sound to the reverberant sound varies depending how far away the listener (microphone) is from the sound source.

This effect is illustrated in Figure 3–6, which shows how the level of the direct sound reduces with increasing distance from the sound source. The level of the direct sound decreases with distance from the sound source due to the inverse square law (see earlier in this section). The decrease in level of the direct sound is shown as a straight line in Figure 3–6 because both axes of the graph are logarithmic (dB on the Y axis and doubling

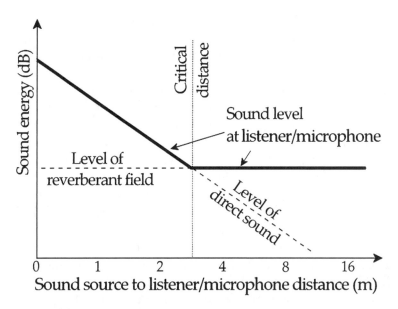

Figure 3–6. *The change in levels of the direct sound and the reverberant field with distance from a source in a room as well as the critical distance.*

of distance as a fixed length on the X axis). The level of the reverberant field remains constant with distance. The point where these two lines intersect occurs at the distance at which the levels of the direct sound and the reverberant field are equal, and this distance is known as the *critical distance*. Every space has its own critical distance that is governed by the reverberant field in that space, which results from the overall amount of sound energy that is absorbed at reflections from the space boundaries or objects within the space. The change in level of the direct sound with distance is the same in any space since it is governed by the inverse square law. When the distance between the listener (or microphone) and the sound source is less than the critical distance, the direct sound dominates, and when they are more than the critical distance apart, the reverberant field dominates. The critical

distance is typically around 0.5 m in a living room and 2 m to 3 m in a large, highly reverberant space such as a cathedral.

Speech intelligibility for a listener in a space depends on the level of the direct sound relative to the level of the reverberant field. Best intelligibility arises when the direct sound dominates; the listener (microphone) is less than the critical distance from the sound source. A useful guideline for keeping speech intelligibility high is to place all the listeners within the critical distance of the sound source. However, this is not, of course, always possible, particularly in a large space designed for big audiences or congregations, such as concert halls, churches, lecture theaters, classrooms, theaters, or opera houses. Large performance spaces are often designed acoustically to have a low reverberation time and therefore a low reverberant field level, which results in a strong direct sound everywhere in the space and a large critical distance.

There are two ways in which intelligibility can be improved within an existing space, either by lowering the reverberation time by modifying the surface materials of a room, or by enhancing the level of the direct sound using an electronic sound reinforcement system. These are dealt with in the following section and Chapter 4, respectively. In the limit, it might appear that a space with no reverberant field would be an ideal acoustic solution (this is how sound is heard in an anechoic room or outside on a still day on a grassy hilltop). However, such a listening situation does not produce a *pleasant* sound to listen to. We need a certain amount of reverberation to be comfortable in our listening. Indeed, the reverberant field has an additional benefit for the speaker or singer, in that it raises the overall acoustic level in the space that arrives at the ears of the listener(s) (see Figure 3–5), thereby ensuring that (a) the sound level is high enough for listening comfort, and (b) the speaker and singer do not have to overly exert their vocal skills. The trick is to use the reverberant field to achieve a balance of intelligibility and listening pleasantness.

MODIFYING THE ACOUSTICS OF A SPACE

Introduction

The acoustics of a space are governed by reflections from surfaces, whether from the walls, floor, ceiling, or objects within the space. The materials from which these surfaces are made control the nature of these reflections in terms of the amount of energy that is absorbed by the surface and therefore the amount that is reflected back into the space; it also depends on whether different frequency components are absorbed by dissimilar amounts. All typical materials that are used in buildings to cover surfaces are subjected to acoustic measurements to determine the amount of acoustic energy that is absorbed at different frequencies spaced one octave apart, usually 125 Hz, 250 Hz, 500 Hz, 1 kHz, 2 kHz, 4 kHz, and 8 kHz. Note that one octave change up (down) is achieved by doubling (halving) the frequency.

The acoustics of a space can be modified by controlling the reflections, and two options are available: (a) the material covering a reflecting surface can be changed, and (b) reflecting surfaces can be moved, removed, or added. The first option can be applied to any existing surface within a space. The second option is rather more limited, since the main boundaries (walls, floor, ceiling) are fixed. However, the introduction of additional reflecting surfaces is a very useful technique for enhancing the sound that is heard by the speaker or singer, thereby enabling better self-monitoring of vocal output. This section provides general practical guidance on the effects that each route can have on the acoustics of a space in the context of a vocal performance.

Acoustics of Surface Materials

The acoustic properties of different surface materials typically used in buildings vary in terms of (a) the amount of acoustic energy they absorb, and (b) how this acoustic absorption changes with frequency. When sound is reflected, a proportion of its energy is absorbed by the reflecting surface, and the remainder is reflected. The amount of acoustic energy absorbed is usually quoted as a value between 0 and 1, where 0 indicates no absorption (all acoustic energy is reflected) and 1 indicates complete absorption (no acoustic energy is reflected). Therefore, if 0.7 (or 70%) of the energy is absorbed, then the remainder (1–0.7) 0.3 (or 30%) is reflected. Tables of acoustic absorption values exist for common building materials at octave spaced frequencies above and below 1 kHz to enable acoustic designers to predict the overall acoustic properties of a space.

Table 3–1 provides acoustic absorption values for a range of common surface materials found in rooms, as well as values for chairs and people. These are not provided as an exhaustive list (full tables run to hundreds of pages); rather, they are included to enable discussion of typical acoustic absorption properties of common classes of surface materials. From the acoustic absorption values given in Table 3–1, it can be seen that surface materials that have small gaps in their surface structure or are acoustically *porous*, such as carpets and curtains, increase absorption at high frequencies; for example, notice how the acoustic absorption effect of heavyweight curtains changes with increasing frequency. More rigid structures that do not have gaps in their surface structure and are acoustically nonporous, such as glass, plasterboard,

Table 3–1. Typical acoustic absorption values for a range of common building materials at octave spaced frequencies above and below 1 kHz

Surface Material	125 Hz	250 Hz	500 Hz	1 kHz	2 kHz	4 kHz
Wooden floorboards on joists	0.15	0.11	0.10	0.07	0.06	0.07
Carpet with underlay	0.08	0.24	0.57	0.69	0.71	0.73
Plaster on lath	0.14	0.10	0.06	0.05	0.04	0.03
Plasterboard	0.29	0.10	0.05	0.04	0.07	0.09
Painted plaster	0.01	0.01	0.02	0.02	0.02	0.02
Wood paneling	0.30	0.25	0.18	0.12	0.07	0.04
Unpainted concrete breeze block	0.36	0.44	0.31	0.29	0.39	0.25
Painted concrete breeze block	0.10	0.05	0.06	0.07	0.09	0.08
Window glass	0.35	0.25	0.18	0.12	0.07	0.04
Lightweight curtains	0.03	0.04	0.11	0.17	0.24	0.35
Heavyweight curtains	0.14	0.35	0.55	0.72	0.70	0.65

or wood paneling, increase absorption at low frequencies; for example, notice the change in acoustic absorption with frequency for window glass.

The reverberation time for a space can be calculated if the volume (V) of the space (*length × width × height*), the acoustic absorption values for each of the surface materials (α_1, α_2, α_3, . . .), and their areas within the space (S_1, S_2, S_3, . . .) are known, using the following equation, known as the *Sabine reverberation time equation*.

$$RT_{60} = \frac{0.61 \times V}{S_1\alpha_1 + S_2\alpha_2 + S_3\alpha_3 + \ldots} \quad (3\text{-}3)$$

Calculating Reverberation Time for a Room

The most convenient way of carrying out this calculation is by using a spreadsheet, but a calculator or pencil and paper can also be used. By way of example, RT_{60} is calculated for an imaginary room of length 4 m, width 3.5 m, and height 2.5 m. The floor is wooden floor-

boards on joists, the ceiling is plaster on lath, the walls are plasterboard, and there are two windows that are each 2.5 m by 1.5 m. Doors are usually ignored in such calculations because their areas are small compared to the total surface area.

Table 3–2 shows how the areas (the values for S_1, S_2, S_3, etc.) are found for this example, and it is worth noting that the windows are part of the walls, and that their area is subtracted from the total wall area to provide S4. The acoustic absorption values (α) are found from Table 3–1, and they are multiplied by their areas to give the values shown in Table 3–3 for each frequency, under the column headings $S\alpha$. These $S\alpha$ values have the unit *Sabin*, after Walter Clement Sabine who proposed equation 3-2 in the 1890s. Using the total for the surface areas multiplied by the acoustic absorption of the surface materials (the row labeled $S_1\alpha1 + S_2\alpha2 + S_3\alpha3 + S_4\alpha4$ for the room in Table 3–3), RT_{60} is calculated using equation 3-3. The volume of this room is 35 m³ (L × W × H = 4 × 3.5 × 2.5 = 35 m³). The resulting RT_{60} is plotted in Figure 3–7.

Table 3–2. Calculation of areas for example room (L = 4 m; W = 3.5 m, H = 2.5 m) as required for reverberation time calculation, where S_1, S_2, S_3, S_4 are the areas of the floor, ceiling, windows, and walls (without the windows), respectively.

	Surface	Material	Area Calculation	Area
S_1	floor	wooden floorboards	L × W: 4 × 3.5	14.0 m²
S_2	ceiling	plaster on lath	L × W: 4 × 3.5	14.0 m²
S_3	windows	glass	2 × (2.5 × 1.5)	7.5 m²
	walls	painted plaster and glass	(L × L × W × W) × H: (4 × 4 × 3.5 × 3.5) × 2.5	37.5 m²
S_4	walls minus windows	painted plaster	37.5 – 7.5	30.0 m²

Table 3–3. Calculation of RT_{60} for sample room, using the areas given in Table 3–2 and the appropriate acoustic absorption values for the surface materials provided in Table 3–1. Three calculations are shown for the room as specified, the room with curtains hung to one and a half times the area of the windows and the room with curtains and fully fitted carpet. Equation 3-3 is used to calculate RT_{60}. The resulting RT_{60} values are plotted graphically in Figure 3–7.

Room ($L = 4\ m; W = 3.5\ m, H = 2.5\ m$)		Area (m^2)	S 125 Hz (Sabins)	S 250 Hz (Sabins)	S 500 Hz (Sabins)	S 1 kHz (Sabins)	S 2 kHz (Sabins)	S 4 kHz (Sabins)
	Surface (material)							
S_1	floor (floorboards)	14	2.10	1.54	1.40	0.98	0.84	0.98
S_2	ceiling (plaster on lath)	14	1.96	1.40	0.84	0.70	0.56	0.42
S_3	windows (glass)	7.5	1.31	0.94	0.68	0.45	0.26	0.15
S_4	walls (plasterboard)	30	0.30	0.30	0.60	0.60	0.60	0.60
$S_1\alpha 1 + S_2\alpha 2 + S_3\alpha 3 + S_4\alpha 4$			5.67	4.18	3.52	2.73	2.26	2.15
RT_{60} (s)			0.99	1.35	1.60	2.06	2.49	2.62

continues

81

Table 3–3. *continued*

Room (L = 4 m; W = 3.5 m, H = 2.5 m)		125 Hz S (Sabins)	250 Hz S (Sabins)	500 Hz S (Sabins)	1 kHz S (Sabins)	2 kHz S (Sabins)	4 kHz S (Sabins)
Surface (material)	Area (m²)						
Room + Curtains							
S_1 floor (floorboards)	14	2.10	1.54	1.40	0.98	0.84	0.98
S_2 ceiling (plaster on lath)	14	1.96	1.40	0.84	0.70	0.56	0.42
S_3 curtains to 1.5 area	7.5	1.58	3.94	6.19	8.10	7.88	7.31
S_4 walls (plasterboard)	30	0.30	0.30	0.60	0.60	0.60	0.60
$S_1\alpha1 + S_2\alpha2 + S_3\alpha3 + S_4\alpha4$		5.94	7.18	9.03	10.38	9.88	9.31
RT_{60} (s)		0.95	0.79	0.62	0.54	0.57	0.61
Room + Curtains + Carpet							
S_1 floor (carpet)	14	2.10	1.54	1.40	0.98	0.84	0.98
S_2 ceiling (plaster on lath)	14	1.96	1.40	0.84	0.70	0.56	0.42
S_3 curtains to 1.5 area	7.5	1.58	3.94	6.19	8.10	7.88	7.31
S_4 walls (plasterboard)	30	0.30	0.30	0.60	0.60	0.60	0.60
$S_1\alpha1 + S_2\alpha2 + S_3\alpha3 + S_4\alpha4$		4.96	9.00	15.61	19.06	18.98	18.55
RT_{60} (s)		1.14	0.63	0.36	0.30	0.30	0.30

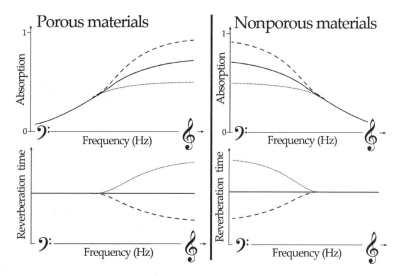

Figure 3–7. *An illustration of the typical acoustic effects of porous and nonporous surface materials on the absorption and reverberation time (RT$_{60}$) of a room (solid lines), and the changes when their areas are increased (dashed lines) or decreased (dotted lines).*

In terms of its surface materials, the sample room is not unlike the bare rooms of a house when one first moves in. The sound of such rooms is very reverberant, particularly at high frequencies, which manifests itself in speech sounds such as /s/ being especially obvious and ringing. In a domestic room, curtains would usually be added over the windows, and a carpet would be placed on the floor. It should be noted that curtains are usually of a greater area than the windows that they cover; they overlap the edges, and they hang in small folds or pleats. This does make a difference in the effect that the curtains will have on the acoustics, and this is accounted for by indicating how much larger the surface area of the curtains is compared with the window they are covering as an area multiplier. In this case, the curtains are assumed to be hung to one and a half times the area of the window, and the factor 1.5 is included in the calculation. The RT$_{60}$ cal-

culation is carried out for the addition of curtains, and again for the addition of curtains and carpet (see Table 3–3), and the resulting RT$_{60}$ values are plotted in Figure 3–7.

The plots of RT$_{60}$ in Figure 3–7 for the addition first of curtains and then of a carpet are very typical. Both curtains and carpet absorb high frequencies to a much greater degree than low frequencies, and this is shown as a large reduction in RT$_{60}$, especially at 1 kHz and above. In a home, our listening preference is for RT$_{60}$ values between about 0.3 and 1 second, and a rise at the low frequency (bass) end, as shown here with the addition of the curtains and carpet, is generally preferred. This example provides a basis for the calculation of RT$_{60}$ for any space, providing the acoustic absorption values are known (these are tabulated in extensive tables for commonly used building materials). The other key reason for the example is to demonstrate that the acoustics of a room can be altered by changing the surface materials in the space.

The relative distribution of acoustically porous and nonporous surfaces within a space determines the reverberation time at different frequencies. Changing this balance provides a means of modifying reverberation time and therefore the reverberant field level within a space. While some modifications would involve structural alterations and are therefore not available for immediate (on the day of the performance) action, the removal or addition of soft furnishing materials such as curtains, rugs, or cushions can make a very significant and acoustically exceedingly useful difference.

Figure 3–7 illustrates the acoustic absorbing effects of porous and nonporous surface materials with frequency (low to high or bass to treble), as well as a fictitious overall reverberation time. It also shows the effect on reverberation time of increasing or decreasing the amount of soft furnishing (porous materials) and nonporous materials within a space. Bear in mind that adding or removing porous materials from a space can be achieved by closing or opening curtains, respectively. Note also that curtains are typically provided to cover a window, and therefore closing the curtains has the double effect of increasing the acoustically porous surface (the curtain itself) *and* decreasing the acoustically nonporous surface (the window's glass), as illustrated in the example calculation detailed in Table 3–3. The acoustic effect of closed curtains can be increased by providing curtains consisting of either more material (multiple folds) or material of a heavier weight, and leaving the curtains partly open offers intermediate possibilities. Curtains

are therefore often used as a straightforward method for acoustic modification, and sometimes curtains are provided in a performance space (and they are not necessarily placed over windows) specifically to enable acoustic modifications to be made.

In practice, changes can be made to the reverberation time of a space to bring it within the range generally considered appropriate for the kind of acoustic material to be performed in it. In practice, values can differ considerably, but typical values are as follows.

- control room: 0.1 s to 0.3 s
- speech: 0.4 s to 1.0 s
- chamber music: 0.8 s to 1.5 s
- orchestral music: 1.0 s to 2.5 s
- church organ and choral music: 1.5 s to 8.0 s

Changing Surface Materials in a Space

A key objective in acoustic design is a reasonably constant reverberation time at all frequencies except at low frequencies, where an increase is generally desirable. It is not within the scope of this book to deal with a full reverberation time design for a room (reading material is listed at the end of the chapter). Rather, it is the main acoustic effects that different materials can have on the acoustics of a space that are presented to enable vocal performers, stage directors, those responsible for buildings, and others to make simple, practical changes to spaces to improve the acoustic experience of performers and their audiences.

The greatest potential for making simple acoustic alterations to improve the vocal performance and listening experience exists for rooms that have not been specifically acoustically designed as performance spaces. In many cases, humans are using their voices on a daily basis in rooms that have been constructed with no consideration having been given to acoustic design, such as many school classrooms, seminar rooms, lecture halls, hotel ballrooms, club back rooms, and church halls. Intelligibility depends on the relative levels of the direct sound and the reverberant field; this and the importance of the critical distance have been introduced in the section Sound Modification by a Space. In terms of a vocal performer, there are two key aspects to consider: (a) how well the performer can monitor her/his own voice, and (b) how comfortably and intelligibly the audience can hear the sound. There are a number of things that can typically be used to improve both these situations in practice, and practical suggestions supported with underlying reasoning are provided below.

PERFORMING TO BEST ACOUSTIC ADVANTAGE IN A SPACE

Introduction

Any performance requires preparation, and since the acoustics of the performance space affect the sound received by the listeners, attention should be paid to achieving the best acoustic result from the space itself. Some time needs to be devoted to this prior to any performance in order to gain familiarity with the acoustics of the space itself, and to consider making changes to its layout. No special equipment is needed but the results can be dramatic in terms of the

overall performance as seen and heard by the audience. The acoustics of the space should be viewed as a tool that is available to the vocal performer. While proper attention to making the space work well acoustically can enhance the final result, using it as offered having gained no familiarity with it in advance can trip up even the best vocal practitioners to the detriment of the final result.

Bearing in mind that the acoustics of a space are determined by the relative positions of the sound source and the listener, it is worth thinking creatively about how a room is laid out for a performance. Even if there is a stage, it is not necessarily the case that that stage is the acoustically optimal place from which to perform. If the audience seating is not fixed, the possibility of moving the seating around should be considered. This is especially important when working in spaces that have not been designed acoustically for optimum vocal performance such as most church halls, school classrooms, seminar rooms, conference breakout rooms, hotel ballrooms, and other spaces where the seating is moveable. When considering where to perform from within a space, however, there are clearly also visual and practical issues to resolve when considering changing the sound source and/or listener position for best acoustic effect.

Different types of music work better acoustically in different spaces, and choral conductors should be aware of this when planning programs to be performed in different venues. Music with much rapid contrapuntal detail will tend to become blurred and the detail lost in a building with a high reverberation time, whereas slow-moving polyphonic music works can be significantly enhanced when performed in spaces with high reverberation times, such as a cathedral.

Acoustic, Visual, and Practical Considerations

Acoustically it is important (see section on Sound Modification by a Space) that (a) the balance between the direct sound and the reverberant field is optimized for intelligibility, pleasantness, and overall loudness, and (b) the performer is able to monitor the output comfortably to combat any tendency towards vocal strain. It is better acoustically to have the audience close to the performers to allow a maximum number to be within the critical distance, thereby providing them with a high direct sound level. If those in the audience who are further away are having difficulty hearing a vocalist, then the acoustic level can be raised by increasing the reverberant field level. This requires an increase in reflected sound, which might be achieved by opening curtains to acoustically expose window glass, or by removing acoustically absorbing surfaces or objects. Conversely, if the sound is too reverberant, which will tend to impair intelligibility particularly for those at the greatest distance from the performers, the reverberant field level can be reduced by closing curtains and/or adding acoustically absorbing surfaces or objects. Such modifications have to be done judiciously, however, to achieve a balance between overall level and intelligibility, noting that this can never be optimal for every member of the audience.

Visually it is important that the performers can be seen clearly by the audience and that the number of blind spots (such as seats with obscured views due to pillars, other members of the audience sitting further forward, or other obstructions) is minimized. It is also essential that the performers can see the audience easily to gain and maintain eye contact, to enable their reaction to be gauged during the performance, and to make appropriate changes as the performance progresses. There may, of course, be issues relating to the lighting to be resolved to ensure that visual contact is two-way. If there are blind spots, it can be useful if the performer moves around whenever possible to help resolve them, but it is worth being aware that movement is likely to create new blind spots elsewhere. A constant awareness of one's audience gained by looking around will keep track of and allow something to be done about full audience inclusion. Bear in mind that a blind spot blocking the view for a member of the audience is also a blind spot preventing the performer from seeing that member of the audience.

Practically, there can be a large acoustic difference in performing from different positions. In many situations it is not feasible to move the audience; perhaps the seating is fixed, there is a stage, podium, or lectern, or regulations state that the fire exit doors have to be at the back, front, or side. However, as a performer there is always the possibility of making an informed decision as to the performance position. The presence of a lectern or podium does not necessarily indicate the optimal position from where to perform; its position has more likely been decided based on overall visual appearance.

Working the Space to Best Acoustic Advantage

Finding a good acoustic position from which to perform can be done by testing the acoustics of the space by moving around it using a handclap as a sound source and listening to the result. A hand-clap is a single, short acoustic sound input to the space, and the sound modifying effect of any space will present the direct sound, early sound, and reverberant sound (see Figure 3–4) to any ear or microphone within the space. One thing to listen out for is flutter echoes, which are best described as a *ping*—a ringing note. If flutter echoes are present, it means that any sound produced by a sound source placed in the position where the handclap was made will be colored by that ping. Flutter echoes occur when the sound source is between two exactly parallel and smooth surfaces, and the resulting sound modification effect is to produce a ping as the sound is trapped between the parallel surfaces, being reflected back and forth. Flutter echoes should be avoided if at all possible; continue moving around the space testing with handclaps to find a spot without them (they are usually localized over quite a small region of sound source positions).

When performing on a stage, it is important to be aware that the stage is acoustically like a small room linked to a larger room (the auditorium). This is particularly the case when there is a proscenium arch at the join and the sound energy levels arriving in the auditorium can be considerably lower than those in the stage area. Once again the best advice is to listen to the space and get to know its sound. Ask a colleague to stand and speak or sing from the performer's position on stage and move around both the stage and the auditorium to obtain a listener's ear view of the sound output from the space in different positions as well as a comparison between the sound energy levels on- and off-stage.

In some situations, background noise can be a serious issue. This is less likely in a space designed for public performances, such as theaters, lecture halls, and opera houses, but relatively high levels of noise are sometimes present in other spaces where one is asked to perform vocally, such as classrooms, church halls, or back rooms in pubs, clubs, or hotels. These are the unwanted sound sources as illustrated in Figure 3–2, and they can either be internal or external. Noise can obscure or mask other sounds, and in the context of speech or singing, certain sounds of the language can be lost to the listener depending on the nature of the noise, thereby compromising intelligibility.

The sounds that are affected by noise will depend on the nature of the noise itself. Noise that is hisslike contains high frequency components and it will tend to mask sounds with high frequency components (see Chapter 2) such as fricatives. Buzzlike noises, such as the drone of electric motors in ventilation or air conditioning systems, will tend to mask frequency components in the formant frequency range, potentially masking vowels. Traffic or aircraft noise tends to cover a wide frequency range and therefore has the potential to mask all sounds. Short bursts of noise, perhaps from hammering, can affect the perception of plosive bursts.

One way to combat noise is to speak or sing at a higher level, but this is not an ideal solution as it places undue strain on the performer's voice. It is worth listening to a space to appreciate the nature of the unwanted noise—it is rare to find a space with no unwanted noise! Sometimes the source of the noise can be turned off. Perhaps a heater or ventilation fan could be turned off at the start of the session, turned on again in the interval, and off again for the second half. If the noise is external, perhaps from traffic or aircraft, then it is worth ensuring that windows are closed properly, noting that if they are required to be open for ventilation, they could be closed at the start of the session, opened in the interval, and closed again for the second half.

The sources of some noises may not be identifiable or may not be locally controllable. Usually a noise will be worse in some parts of the space, and if this can be identified by careful listening, there may be scope for changing the layout of the room to avoid any noise hot spots. One other form of noise that cannot be checked beforehand is that produced by the audience. Have a strategy thought out for dealing with audience noise such as chatter, mobile telephones, or late arrivals. Raising the performance level to combat such noises rarely works since the noise levels will often be raised also, and this does have an acoustic energy cost that could result in vocal problems if it becomes a persistent habit. One method that can work very well is silence—a silent pause accompanied with a stare towards the noise source can be most effective and it has no acoustic energy cost!

Vocal Performance Considerations

A key element of vocal performance, whether singing or speaking, is communication of the text. The acoustic effect of the space can serve to destroy all endeavors to annunciate consonants carefully, because the overall sound reaching the ears of listeners who are well beyond the critical distance (see Sound Modification by a Space) is "blurred" or "mushy," so that the acoustic detail that is important for distinguishing between individual sounds is lost, with the result that the message becomes very difficult to understand.

Figure 3–8 illustrates this effect in terms of how reverberation serves to extend individual sounds acoustically in time, and the potential there is for them to overlap. The figure shows the average pressure level of the two consonants in the word *beat* (SAMPA: /bit/), for the situations where /b/ is louder than /t/ and /t/ is louder than /b/. The reverberation decay is indicated for a short and a long reverberation time (RT_{60}); this is how the energy of each consonant would decay. Notice that the later consonant is the one that could be obscured or masked by the reverberant decay of the first, and that this is the case for the long RT_{60} shown. When the later consonant /t/ is louder than the first /b/, complete masking cannot occur. Deliberate articulation of final consonants is therefore particularly important in highly reverberant spaces to combat this effect and ensure that the listener is provided with the acoustic cues required to enable all sounds to be heard clearly and identified. In addition, shortening individual syllables or sounds and lengthening the gaps between them will make space to allow the reverberation to die away before the next acoustic event.

One of the less well understood and compensated for acoustic issues facing anyone using his voice regularly in front of a group of people is the extent to which he can hear himself adequately. This is vitally important, because our vocal output is continuously being monitored by our brain, known as *self-*

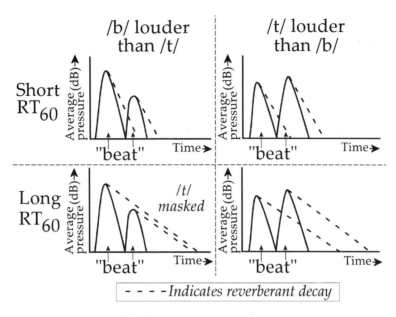

Figure 3–8. *Illustration of the potential masking effect of a short and a long reverberation time (RT$_{60}$) on the second consonant /t/ in beat (SAMPA: /bit/) by the first consonant /b/, depending on their relative levels.*

monitoring. If the acoustic energy level reaching our ears is insufficient, the brain insists that we speak louder so that it can carry out its monitoring job effectively. This is what triggers a tendency to speak or sing louder than is comfortable (and often louder than is actually necessary as far as the audience is concerned), and therein is a common route to vocal strain or more serious vocal problems. This is particularly an issue for those such as teachers or lecturers who use their voices over long periods. Teachers are the largest group presenting for medical attention relating to vocal issues such as strain, laryngitis, or hoarseness. So often, the cause is simply an inability to self-monitor adequately.

Increasing the level of the direct sound that is fed back to the ears of the performer can help to sort this issue out, and this can be achieved in a relatively straightforward manner. Starting with an awareness of the issue, creative possibilities can be thought through to improve matters through the use of acoustically reflecting surfaces placed close to the performer to provide *foldback*. Such reflectors are usually placed behind the performer, so that they are not only of benefit to the performer, but they also enhance the overall sound level that reaches the audience.

Specially made reflectors do exist, but there are ways of moving towards improving foldback using existing materials or apparatus. Any hard surface, such as a white board or blackboard, will serve as an acoustic reflector to provide foldback, and often these are on wheels and can be readily moved. Acoustic screens are becoming increasingly available for use in orchestras and music groups to shield the ears of players sitting in front of loud instruments (e.g., percussion and brass) following renewed concerns about overall sound levels in public spaces. In some areas (in the United Kingdom this last occurred in April 2006), the maximum levels allowed have been lowered, prompting the provision of acoustic screens on health and safety grounds. Where such screens, which are usually made of thick acrylic and mounted on wheels, are available, try them out as reflectors to enhance what the performer is hearing.

When a reflector is set up to provide foldback to the performer, it is important to ensure that the delay involved is not too great. Delay will be incurred because the path travelled by the acoustic wave from the performer to the reflector and back to the performer's ears takes time, which can be determined from the velocity of sound (usually taken as 344 meters per second—see Chapter 1). A delay of no more than about 25 ms will typically not interfere with the benefits provided by the foldback, and in that time sound can travel 8.6 m. (The velocity of sound is 344 meters per second, so in 25 ms [or 0.25 s], sound will travel a distance equal to the time multiplied by the velocity, which is $344 \times 0.25 = 8.6$ m.) Remembering that the sound has to get to the reflector and back, this means that a foldback reflector should be placed within 4.3 m (half of 8.6 m) of the performer. In a small room, there is likely to be at least one wall within 4.3 m of the performer that will serve to provide foldback. However, in a large hall there probably will not be a surface that is close enough to act as a foldback reflector, and that is when it is worth setting up a local reflector.

When working on stage with scenery, it is worth being aware of the potential benefit of improving foldback, especially when performing a major speech, song, or aria. If a speaker is suffering unanticipated vocal strain or a singer is experiencing unexpected tuning difficulties, this could be due to a lack of an appropriate foldback level. With the director's agreement (or instruction), they could perhaps be positioned within 4.3 m of a piece of scenery that could provide acoustic foldback, or perhaps the scenery could be appropriately added to or rearranged.

The importance of foldback has been known to professional pop groups for a long time. Vocal performers are provided with local loudspeakers to provide an appropriate mix of the overall sound output as foldback, which includes their own vocal output. These loudspeakers are usually placed on the stage, so as not to be visually intrusive, with their loudspeakers facing upwards at 45 degrees towards the ears of the performer to localize the sound. Due to the shape of the loudspeaker cases, they are often referred to as *wedges*. Alternatively, foldback can be provided directly into the ears of vocal performers via bud earphones. This is known as *in ear monitoring* and it is especially useful for performers who move around a lot. For vocalists, it is vital that the foldback balance of relative levels of the different instruments and their own vocal output is appropriate. Good working relationships between whoever is in charge, the sound team, and the vocalists are an important part of vocal care in such situations.

When performing with acoustic instrument accompaniment, it is important to ensure that the accompaniment can be heard comfortably to maintain intonation and a proper balance for both performers and audience. It is always worth moving around to find the best position acoustically, and then to consider how that position might be modified to provide best visual presentation to the audience. Often, just a small repositioning can make a huge difference to the overall acoustic coherence of a performance while also serving to provide less chance of problems for vocalists.

SUMMARY

This chapter has introduced sound transmission in a space from the sound source to the microphone or ear of the listener. The concepts of direct sound, early sound, and reverberant sound enable the nature of the sound output from a space to be better understood in terms of how this output sound changes for different sound source or listener positions in a space, and the possibilities that exist for practical and inexpensive acoustic modifications that might be made to a space.

When performing as a vocalist in a space, it is essential to remember that the acoustics of the space itself are a part of the performance. The acoustics of the space should be used to best advantage. Performance spaces are often well set up acoustically, and often there is little choice as to the performance position. Everyday work spaces are rarely set up acoustically, and there are a number of things that can be considered that can make it easier both for listeners to comprehend the message and for the performer's voice. Any use of the voice in any job is a performance. Considering it as such while taking advantage of the advice given herein has the potential not only to improve the quality of vocal life,

but also to gain esteem from those observing the performance. You only have one voice; look after it and use it well.

FURTHER READING

Acoustics of Spaces

Beranek, L. L. (1954). *Acoustics*. New York: McGraw-Hill.

Howard, D. M., & Angus, J. A. S. (2001). Room acoustics: How they affect vocal production and perception. In P. H. Dejonckere (Ed.), *Occupational voice—Care and cure* (pp. 29–46). The Hague, Netherlands: Kugler.

Howard, D. M., & Angus, J. A. S. (2006). *Acoustics and psychoacoustics* (3rd ed.). Oxford, UK: Focal Press.

Modifying the Acoustics of a Space

Everest, F. A. (1984). *The master handbook of acoustics*. TAB Books.

Everest, F. A. (1989). *Acoustic techniques for home and studio* (2nd ed.). TAB Books.

Howard, D. M., & Angus, J. A. S. (2006). *Acoustics and psychoacoustics* (3rd ed.) Oxford, UK: Focal Press.

Performing to Best Advantage in a Space

Howard, D. M., & Angus, J. A. S. (2001). Room acoustics: How they affect vocal production and perception. In P. H. Dejonckere (Ed.), *Occupational voice—Care and cure* (pp. 29–46). The Hague, Netherlands: Kugler.

Potter, J. (2001). *The Cambridge companion to singing*. Cambridge, UK: Cambridge University Press.

Smith, B., & Sataloff, R. T. (2000). *Choral pedagogy*. San Diego, CA: Singular.

CHAPTER 4

Audio System Fundamentals

It is highly likely that at some point in their career, the vocal performer and professional voice user will be required to work with some form of microphone, and therefore they should consider the impact that this, and related audio technology, might have on the vocal source. This chapter introduces audio system fundamentals in terms of sound recording and sound reinforcement technology. The most important element of this audio signal path, from vocal performer through to studio/PA loudspeaker as shown in Figure 4–1, will be considered first of all—the microphone.

Understanding the fundamental operating principles of the device whose responsibility—more than anything else —will determine how the voice will sound when reproduced via another medium is critical to the professional vocalist. This applies equally to either the singing or speaking voice. The basics of how a microphone works will be covered in some detail together with how these principles affect the quality of the vocal pickup. This knowledge can then be used to help influence microphone choice when faced with particular vocal capture scenarios.

Once converted to an electrical signal by the microphone, the voice is ready to be subjected to the wide palette of audio processing options offered by the modern recording studio. The organization and operation of a typical studio mixing desk is introduced, together with how the vocal signal is best conditioned and ready to be recorded to an appropriate medium. The most common and important studio effects are also covered, with guidelines offered for their best use, as well as an overview of the role of the actual recording system and its integration into the wider studio setup. Finally, this chapter considers vocal amplification and sound reinforcement, where the goal is not to make a permanent record of a vocal performance, but rather to present it to a wider audience using an appropriate sound reinforcement system. Three basic setups are considered, together with a guide to live front-of-house and monitor sound mixing and useful troubleshooting steps that can be followed to avoid common problems such as feedback.

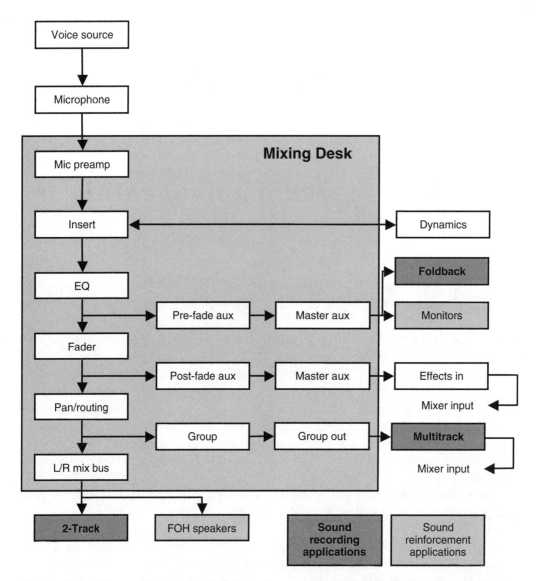

Figure 4–1. *The audio signal path from voice source via mixing desk to destination for both sound recording and sound reinforcement applications.*

MICROPHONES

Introduction

The critical stage in any vocal recording, be it speech or singing, is in the initial capture of the acoustic energy emanat-

ing from the voice source. This acoustic signal is then converted into an equivalent electrical signal that can be stored on an appropriate medium for later playback and further editing and manipulation. In a recording studio the microphones are often considered the most important element in the audio recording chain as they are required to capture a large range of acoustic sound sources (not just voice) and convert them to such an electrical signal suitable for processing by a wide range of audio equipment. Hence, there are many different microphones available to the recording engineer and they can vary greatly in both price and sound. In this case the "sound" of the microphone can refer to the general quality of the audio signal in purely objective terms such as frequency response, distortion, or signal-to-noise ratio. It can also refer to the general perceptual quality of the recorded audio—e.g., warm, bright, harsh, muffled. Some microphones are therefore favored over others for the particular character that they can impart to a recorded voice (in this case), and so the most expensive microphone is not always the best one for the job. It should also be mentioned that the range of microphones available also varies with the application for which they are designed. For instance, a vocal microphone for studio recording would usually be very different from that used for live performance, location film dialogue recording, or television studio and broadcast work. With such a wealth of options to select from it is important to be able to make an informed decision as to what microphone should be used for a specific task. However, in general the following might be required of a typical "good" microphone:

- A flat frequency response
- A good sound
- Low noise, particularly for very quiet sounds
- Low levels of distortion, particularly for very loud sounds
- The ability to deal with both of these extremes—a wide dynamic range

- An appropriate response to sounds from different directions—is it important to pick up sound from all around the microphone, or just those emanating from a single direction?

There are no rigid correlations between any of these factors; no microphone can do everything and all designs have their own inherent limitations. However, it is possible to classify microphones by their basic design, physical characteristics, and the associated properties that arise as a consequence. Hence, what follows is a basic understanding of how a microphone works, and how this design will act to affect the quality of a captured or recorded vocal sound.

Dynamic vs. Condenser

Dynamic microphones (sometimes called moving-coil microphones), as shown in Figure 4–2, are passive and hence have no on-board electronics to boost the signal level, and work on the basis of a varying magnetic field. The microphone consists of a light diaphragm usually made of a plastic material called *Mylar*, coupled to a small copper coil suspended in a permanent magnetic field. When an acoustic pressure wave from a sound source is incident on the microphone capsule, the diaphragm moves backwards and forwards sympathetically. The motion of the coil in the fixed magnetic field induces a voltage, v, across the coil that corresponds to the pressure acting on the diaphragm. This process is called *electromagnetic induction* and is the same principle that is used in loudspeakers.

Dynamic microphones use essentially the same design as a loudspeaker except they convert an acoustic source into an electrical signal rather than con-

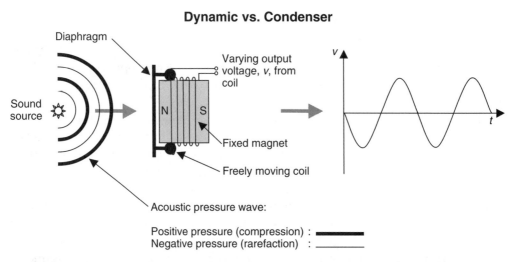

Figure 4–2. *The basic design and functionality of a dynamic microphone.*

verting from the electrical to the acoustic domain. It is also possible to connect a loudspeaker to the input of a mixing desk and use it as a very simple microphone. However, with a loudspeaker, the diaphragm, or speaker cone in this case, and the magnet/coil assembly are much larger and heavier than those found in a microphone capsule, and so they are considerably less sensitive to low level sounds. Loudspeakers are sometimes used to record the bass drum on a drum kit, as they are capable of capturing the very low frequency aspect of this particular sound source in a way that no microphone can.

A variation on the dynamic microphone design is used in *ribbon microphones,* where instead of using a diaphragm and coil combination, a thin and usually corrugated metal ribbon is suspended in a magnetic field. This ribbon moves directly according to the sound waves incident upon it.

Microphones that use the variable capacitor principle are usually called *condenser microphones,* use active electron-

ics, and work on the basis of a varying electric field. In this design, shown in Figure 4–3, the freely moving diaphragm is conductive and has another fixed plate spaced closely behind it separated by a layer of conductive insulation. These two plates are charged or *polarized* with static electricity forming a capacitor. With a capacitor the voltage, v, across plates will vary according to the distance between them. Hence, as the diaphragm moves sympathetically according to the incident acoustic pressure waves, the distance between the plates is varied as is; the capacitance between the plates. This again results in an electrical signal that corresponds directly to the original acoustic pressure wave.

Most modern condenser microphones are of the *electret* type—that is, the plates of the capacitor are permanently prepolarized. Non-electrets require additional electronic circuitry within the microphone housing to charge the plates of the capacitors. Both types of condenser also require an additional preamp stage, again within the microphone housing, to

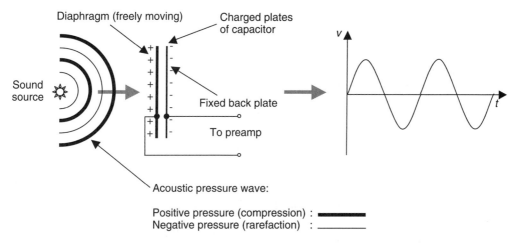

Figure 4–3. *The basic design and functionality of a condenser microphone.*

convert the very high electrical imped-ance of the capacitor to an appropriate low value so that the signal can be eas-ily transmitted down a standard micro-phone cable without too many losses.

The additional circuitry for the inter-nal preamp means that condenser micro-phones require some form of power, either from an internal battery or more commonly via a 48 v dc source called *phantom power*, usually supplied from the mixing desk they are connected to. If the condenser microphone is a non-electret type, it will also require power to charge the plates of the capacitor.

The comparative qualities of dynamic, ribbon, and condenser microphones due to their design and construction can be summarized generally as follows:

Dynamic microphones:
- A relatively thick diaphragm attached to a coil of some mass makes the microphone less sensitive to low level signals (not enough energy to cause the diaphragm to move) and high frequency signals (often having less energy than low frequencies).

- This design acts to color the recorded sound, particularly in the upper-mid and high frequency region.
- The design is good for high volume levels.
- Low sensitivity results in a low output level, requiring more gain to be applied at the mixing desk input, increasing the potential for added noise.
- Low sensitivity implies there is a low level of performer handling noise if a microphone stand is not used.
- The diaphragm/coil combination implies there is a poor transient response—it takes some time for the diaphragm/coil to move, meaning that short, sharp sounds are often not picked up accurately.
- Simple design, with no active elec-tronics, means dynamic microphones are cheap, robust, and reliable, with-standing heat, cold, and humidity.

Ribbon microphones:
- Thin, light diaphragm implies the microphone is very sensitive to low level sounds.

■ The microphone will respond well to high frequencies, again because of the light diaphragm.

■ Very low signal level output, requiring more gain at the mixing desk, potentially resulting in more added noise.

■ Very delicate in operation, again due to the sensitive nature of the design.

Condenser microphones:

■ The diaphragm is light, making the design more sensitive than a dynamic but less sensitive than a ribbon microphone.

■ The design is good for low level and high frequency sounds.

■ Frequency response is wide, extended, and generally more linear with a detailed and clear sound.

■ Transient response is good.

■ It requires battery or external phantom powering.

■ More delicate construction than a dynamic and additional electronic circuitry implies they must be treated with care and can be susceptible to environmental considerations.

■ High output level means less gain required at mixing desk input and so

they often have a good low noise floor.

Microphone Directivity Patterns

Microphones can also be classified according to their *polar pickup* or *directivity pattern*, that is, how sensitive they are to sounds arriving from different directions. Most types of microphones fall into one of two categories:

■ Pressure microphones (omnidirectional)

■ Pressure difference microphones (unidirectional)

Omnidirectional

Figure 4–4(a) shows the basic omnidirectional pattern in a representation known as a *polar plot*. With the front of the microphone capsule placed at the center of the plot, the thick black outer line demonstrates how the signal level at the microphone output varies with the direction of the source. In the case of an omnidirectional microphone there is no variation and the signal level is constant across all angles. Figure 4–4(b) shows

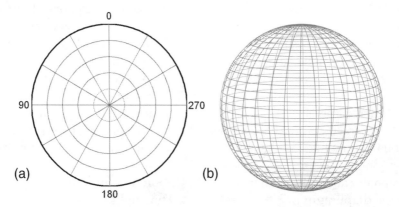

Figure 4–4. *Omnidirectional directivity pattern: (a) 2D polar response; (b) ideal 3D directivity pattern.*

the corresponding three-dimensional directivity pattern. The omnidirectional pattern is achieved by restricting sound entry into the microphone capsule to a single point at the front of the diaphragm, resulting in very little distinction between sound source directions and therefore ensuring a uniform response. Note that Figure 4–4 shows the ideal microphone response, and the reality is not usually so perfect. In particular, at very high frequencies, there will be some departure from this ideal pattern due to the physical size of the microphone capsule providing an acoustical obstruction, and the microphone will show a preference for sounds arriving from the front, although for most applications this will be negligible.

Figure-of-Eight

In this case, the microphone diaphragm is open on both sides and the signal is dependent on the pressure difference or gradient between the two sides. By way of comparison, an omnidirectional microphone is sometimes also called a *pressure microphone* as it responds to the sound pressure level incident on the diaphragm. A pressure difference microphone such as the figure-of-eight is sometimes called a *velocity microphone* as the pressure difference or gradient gives a measure of the velocity of the incident acoustic signal. This gives a bidirectional figure-of-eight response as shown in Figure 4–5. Sound waves incident on the microphone from the front (0 degrees), also known as *on-axis*, or rear (180 degrees) will cause a difference in pressure between both sides of the diaphragm and hence the diaphragm will move accordingly. A pressure wave arriving from behind will produce opposite movement to a pressure wave arriving at the front and so is said to be *out of phase* or *phase reversed*. For a sound wave incident from 90 degrees or 270 degrees, the pressure at the front and rear will be equal, the pressure difference will be zero, and so the diaphragm will not move. A figure-of-eight microphone is said to effectively reject sounds at ± 90 degrees to the frontal axis.

Cardioid

This pattern, so named due its inverted heart shape as shown in Figure 4–6, was

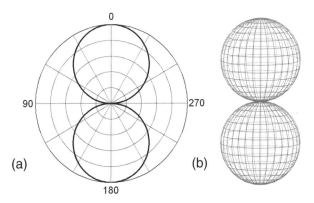

Figure 4–5. *Figure-of-eight directivity pattern: (a) 2D polar response; (b) ideal 3D directivity pattern.*

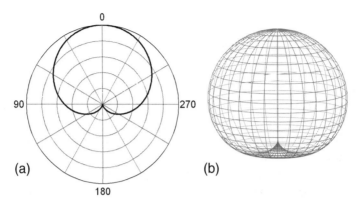

Figure 4–6. *Cardioid directivity pattern: (a) 2D polar response; (b) ideal 3D directivity pattern.*

originally obtained by summing a figure-of-eight capsule and an omnidirectional capsule but is now generally designed using *acoustical resistance* (also called an *acoustic* or *internal labyrinth*). As with the figure-of-eight microphone, the diaphragm is open to sound on both sides. However, acoustical resistance at the rear of the diaphragm is designed to ensure that a signal arriving from 180 degrees is sufficiently delayed so that it arrives at both front and rear simultaneously despite having to travel the extra distance around to the front of the microphone. With the same signal in phase at the front and back of the diaphragm, the pressure difference will be zero, and hence sound from the rear of the microphone is effectively rejected. This has an importance consequence for vocalists using microphones in combination with public address (PA) systems in a live performance, as will be explored in the section Vocal Sound Reinforcement. Typically, a cardioid microphone will provide 20–25 dB of attenuation or rejection for a sound source arriving from the rear for the mid frequency range, compared with a signal on-axis at 0 degrees. The directivity pattern between 0 and 180 degrees varies between these

two extremes, giving the classic cardioid shape that can be seen in Figure 4–6. Again, this is the ideal response, whereas at very low frequencies, the polar pattern tends more to the omnidirectional case, and at very high frequencies a rear lobe develops, resulting in a shape closer to that of a hypercardioid.

Supercardioid and Hypercardioid

These microphone directivity types are variations on the basic cardioid pattern and are often useful for certain applications. If the acoustical resistance path length is varied somewhat from the basic cardioid design, the angle of maximum rejection can be varied and shifted away from 180 degrees. The advantage of these designs is a more focused frontal region, at the expense of a lobe developing at 180 degrees, giving increased signal level for sounds from the rear. This can clearly be seen in the supercardioid polar pickup patterns shown in Figure 4–7. Typically, a cardioid microphone has a useful frontal region, or *acceptance angle* (defined as an angular range ± 0 degrees for which the level of an on-axis sound source varies by no more than ± 3 dB) of about ± 65 degrees either side of the frontal axis. This reduces to approxi-

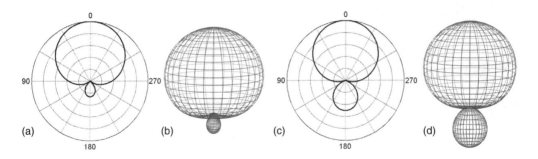

Figure 4–7. *Cardioid family directivity patterns: (a) supercardioid 2D polar response; (b) supercardioid ideal 3D directivity pattern; (c) hypercardioid 2D polar response; (d) hypercardioid ideal 3D directivity pattern.*

mately ± 57 degrees for a supercardioid and ± 52 degrees for a hypercardioid. The cardioid family also has better *reach* than an omnidirectional microphone. This means that in a noisy or reverberant environment, a cardioid type microphone will reject more of this background noise in favor of a sound source at 0 degrees. This leads to the definition of *directivity index* and *distance factor* that help to characterize the cardioid family further.

Assume first of all that an omnidirectional microphone is placed directly in front of a sound source in a noisy environment at a measured distance, *d*. This will serve as a reference from which the directivity index and distance factor can be measured. If a cardioid microphone is then used in the same situation, so that the balance between source and background sound is equivalent to the omnidirectional case, the microphone-to-source distance would be $1.7 \times d$. The supercardioid would be placed at a distance of $1.9 \times d$ and the hypercardioid would be placed at $2.0 \times d$. The multiplying factor in these examples is the distance factor for the microphone.

If the particular cardioid family microphone is now placed at the same

distance as the omnidirectional reference microphone, the balance between source and background sound can be measured in decibels. Hence, with the cardioid pattern, background sounds will be attenuated by 4.8 dB compared with the direct sound from the source. With the supercardioid the attenuation is 5.8 dB and with the hypercardioid, 6 dB. This dB measure is called the directivity index.

Clearly there is an advantage to using a cardioid pattern microphone over an omnidirectional one when recording the voice in non-ideal conditions. The additional advantage with the super- and hypercardioid variants is that a similar sound level and rejection of background noise can be recorded with the microphone placed at a greater distance. This gives the sound engineer some additional flexibility and control in situations where close-miking may not be possible, for instance in live performance.

Supercardioid microphones are also often used in the design of highly directional microphones called *rifle*, *line*, or *shotgun* microphones. These microphones have a long interference tube in front of the main capsule that acts to give a significantly more directional response at upper-mid and high frequencies. With the microphone pointed at a source at 0 degrees, the direct sound will pass directly down the interference tube to the capsule as normal. Sounds that arrive off axis, such as background noise or reverberation, are partially cancelled out by the effect of the interference tube. The length of the tube will determine how effective and directional the microphone is, with a longer tube extending the useful frequency range of the microphone's directional response. The design complexity of these microphones does mean that the directional characteristic is less than ideal across the frequency range. There is some considerable variation, including the development of side lobes, in addition to the desired narrow frontal directivity pattern, and the significant rear lobe that is a consequence of the basic supercardioid capsule that is used.

Although not useful in the recording studio, shotgun microphones do have some specific applications such as in theater PAs, where they are often used across the front of the stage area, and most commonly for field recording on film/television production. In this example good vocal capture is clearly very important, but microphones must be kept out of shot, and hence a highly directional characteristic with good rejection of ambient noise is desirable.

Microphone Frequency Response

So far the basic operating principles of a microphone have been discussed, in terms of how they convert an acoustic signal to an electrical one, and how they respond to a sound arriving from a particular direction. Both of these considerations have a significant impact on how the microphone will actually sound—in theory a microphone should transparently transmit the acoustic signal to the electrical domain without altering its timbre. In practice this is impossible, although in some cases the timbral change that is a consequence is actually a desirable property. The influence a particular microphone might have on the timbre of an on-axis sound source, or how it will impart its own characteristics onto this source, is quantified by its *frequency response*. This is a graph, shown in Figure 4–8, of frequency against signal

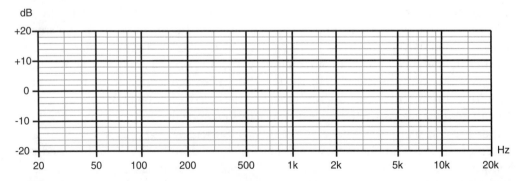

Figure 4–8. *The frequency response graph. The x-axis is a logarithmic scale showing frequency in Hz across the audible range from 20 Hz to 20 kHz. The y-axis is a linear scale in dB showing the change in gain, as it varies with frequency, with positive values denoting signal boost, and negative values denoting signal attenuation.*

level that will be included as part of the data sheet or specifications that come with any microphone.

If a microphone was a truly transparent transducer from the acoustic to electrical domain the corresponding frequency response graph would look like that presented in Figure 4–9. The microphone would neither boost nor attenuate any frequency across the entire audible range from 20 Hz to 20 kHz.

Due to its simple operating principle and low mass diaphragm a typical omnidirectional condenser microphone might demonstrate a frequency response that is generally considered to be flat, except at the very lowest and highest frequencies, as shown in Figure 4–10.

By way of contrast, the frequency response of a typical cardioid dynamic microphone, a type commonly used for vocal work, is often very nonlinear. An example is shown in Figure 4–11. There are two points to notice from this graph. First of all, the attenuation at either end of the response is present as in Figure 4–10 but has a more significant roll-off. At the low end this starts at about 200 Hz and at the high end this starts at about 10 kHz. In the latter case this

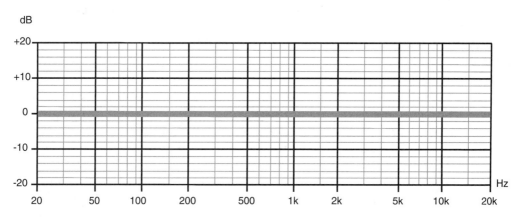

Figure 4–9. *The frequency response of an ideal microphone, denoted by the thick grey line. In this example it neither boosts nor attenuates any particular frequency, being truly transparent to the sound source.*

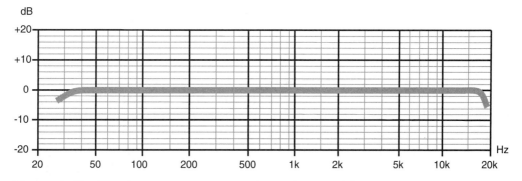

Figure 4–10. *The frequency response of a typical omnidirectional condenser microphone. It is almost exactly flat except for an attenuation (or roll-off) at the highest and lowest frequencies.*

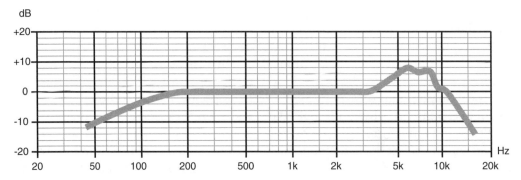

Figure 4–11. *The frequency response of a typical cardioid dynamic microphone. There is significant roll-off below about 200 Hz and above 10 kHz. Note also the peak in the 5–10 kHz range.*

is due to the significant mass of the diaphragm/coil combination making the microphone less sensitive to high frequency signal components that typically have less energy. The second aspect is the clear peak in the response in the 5–10 kHz range, often called a *presence peak*; this is a designed characteristic of the microphone. The low frequency roll-off is also a designed characteristic of the microphone, due to what is known as *proximity effect*, being a consequence of the pressure difference principle that all cardioid family microphones are based on.

Proximity effect is the bass boost evident when a cardioid microphone is used in close proximity to the sound source. The effect is also evidenced with other pressure difference microphones, although it is most pronounced with the cardioid design. Microphone designers often make good use of this proximity effect to help flatten the overall frequency response, as in the example shown in Figure 4–11. A microphone with this property is designed to be placed close to the source, and if proximity effect is not accounted for in this way in the overall frequency response, the micro-

phone will usually incorporate a high-pass/low-cut filter, often with a variable cutoff point, to compensate for this bass boost. Proximity effect can also make a cardioid microphone very sensitive to handling noises and to the effects of wind. Figure 4–12 shows the frequency response of two microphones now taking proximity effect into account. Figure 4–12(a) is the cardioid dynamic microphone from Figure 4–11, now with additional information relating to the low end response at various distances from the on-axis source. Figure 4–12(b) is the frequency response of a typical cardioid condenser microphone with a flat frequency response, with additional information given to demonstrate the effect on the frequency response of the built-in high-pass filter designed to minimize proximity effect when positioned close to the sound source.

The frequency response of a microphone will also depend on the size of the diaphragm. The larger the diaphragm, the more efficient it is at transducing low frequencies and less efficient at high frequencies. Finally, when considering the frequency response of a microphone,

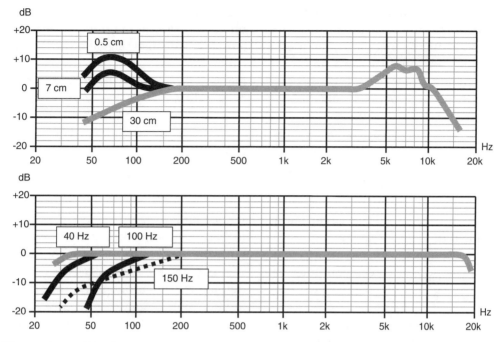

Figure 4–12. *The frequency response of two microphones incorporating proximity effect compensation. (a) Cardioid dynamic microphone at three distances from an on-axis sound source. The closer the microphone is to the source, the more pronounced the bass boost effect, compensating for the standard low frequency roll-off at distance. (b) A cardioid condenser designed with a flat frequency response. A variable high-pass filter is used to compensate for proximity effect when used close to the source.*

the presented graphs, as often found on any microphone data sheet, are generally only true for an on-axis (0 degrees) sound source. So it is important with non-omnidirectional microphones to ensure that they are positioned carefully and correctly to make the best use of their characteristics. With the source off-axis to the microphone, the result can sound colored and not ideal. This is even more important with shotgun microphones where off-axis sounds, a moving sound source, or even reflections from surfaces within the recording environment can result in phase cancellations that will produce peaks or nulls in the ideal frequency response of the microphone.

Other Important Microphone Considerations

Sensitivity

The sensitivity of a microphone is determined by placing it in front of a reference sound source with a measured sound pressure level (SPL) of 94 dB at 1 kHz. This value for SPL is the same as a pressure value of 1 Pa. The unloaded output voltage of the microphone is then measured, giving its sensitivity value. Generally this is quoted in mV/PA as the measured voltage is actually low, or may alternatively be given in dBV. In general, a condenser microphone will have a higher level of sensitivity than a similar dynamic microphone; however, the intended use must also be considered. Dynamic microphones are often used in very close proximity to the sound source and so the average output will be somewhat increased. Condenser microphones are often used at some distance from the source, and in some cases at many meters distant, and so ultimately they will result in a comparable signal level to a close-up dynamic microphone. Large diaphragm microphones also generally have a higher sensitivity rating, as the larger surface area makes the microphone more sensitive to changes in acoustic pressure, hence developing a greater output signal.

Noise

The inherent noise or self-noise of a microphone is the measured output level when the microphone is isolated from all other sound sources. Typically this is given in units of dBA, which refers to a dB SPL measure that is then A-weighted to account for how our hearing mechanism is sensitive to, and hence varies with, frequency. So, if a microphone has a self-noise level of 20 dBA, this is equivalent to a theoretically ideal microphone placed in a room with a stated noise level of 20 dBA. *Signal-to-noise ratio* is a quantity defined as the ratio between the noise level of a medium and a signal transmitted through this medium. For a microphone the signal used is typically a 1 kHz tone at 94 dB SPL (1 Pa). So for the previous example, with a self-noise measure of 20 dBA, the signal-to-noise ratio would be 74 dB, effectively measuring the signal level above the noise floor normalized to 0 dB. Therefore, as large diaphragm microphones generally have a higher sensitivity, and a greater output level, they will also have a better signal-to-noise ratio. Ultimately, the higher the signal level from the microphone, due to design, inherent characteristics, or acoustic signal level, the less gain that needs to be applied at the mixing desk input, and so the less additional noise will added to the original signal. The mixing desk and other recording equipment considerations will be discussed in the next section.

Maximum Acceptable Level or Overload Point

If noise and sensitivity give a measure as to how well a microphone will behave with the quietest of signals, the maximum acceptable level or overload point defines the microphone characteristics at very high (= loud) signal levels. The effective upper limit in dB SPL that a microphone can deal with is determined by measuring the harmonic distortion present in the output signal. Typically, a dynamic microphone may quote a maximum acceptable level of 156 db SPL for less than 3% distortion. This level of distortion may be inaudible, and so more important is the overload point or clipping level of the microphone that will be particularly noticeable on high amplitude peaks in the signal, often associated with fast transient-type sounds. This clipping point is caused by the diaphragm reaching its maximum limit of displacement point, or the preamplifier electronic circuits being overloaded. It is very audible and unpleasant sounding and should be avoided at all costs.

Finally, with the maximum acceptable level and noise floor of a microphone defined, the *dynamic range* can be quoted as being the difference in dB SPL between these two quantities and the useful variation between the quietest and loudest acoustic signals that a microphone can reasonably deal with.

General Tips for Microphone Use

- Always use stands that give good stability and allow the microphone to be raised to as high a level as required.
- Use shock mounts if they are available to prevent noise from vibration, or place the stands on some rubber or sponge mats (carpet tiles can also be useful).
- Keep microphone cables tidy and away from where they might be stepped on or tripped over. Allow some cable slack at the bottom of the microphone stand to allow for easy repositioning or to minimize accidental tripping.
- Check that any filters or level controls on the microphone capsules themselves are set appropriately, or left in bypass mode. If using two microphones—perhaps for stereo— make sure both are set the same.
- Do not use the foam shields often supplied with microphones as this can attenuate high frequency detail. If recording outside, perhaps for broadcast work, high quality wind shields should be used instead.
- If microphones need batteries for phantom powering, always make sure they are checked and replaced as necessary before a session. Have spares ready also, just in case.

Microphone Summary

From what has been presented so far, it is clear that there are a great many factors that must be considered when selecting a microphone for a specific recording task. Making an informed microphone choice for vocal recording or performance will be considered in more detail in Chapter 5, but this section is concluded with a summary by polar pickup pattern.

Omnidirectional

- Simple operation and design— a pressure microphone.
- Wide, flat, extended frequency response.
- Good pickup of both low and high frequencies.
- Will also capture much of the reverberation present in the recording environment.
- Poor isolation from other sounds unless the microphone is close to the sound source.
- Not affected by proximity effect.

Cardioid Family

- More complex operation and design —a pressure difference or velocity microphone.
- Good rejection of reverberation and background noise.
- Good isolation from other sound sources.
- Proximity effect is a rise in relative level of bass frequencies.
- Cardioid has the widest front angle pickup and the best rear rejection.
- Supercardioid has more isolation than a cardioid and less reverberation pickup.
- Hypercardioid has the most side rejection, isolation, and rejection in terms of reverberation, background noise, and other sound sources.

Figure of Eight

- A simple pressure difference or velocity microphone—no need to be designed with phase cancellation in mind for acoustic null points.

■ Good front and rear pickup with maximum rejection of sounds arriving from the sides.

VOICE RECORDING SYSTEMS

Introduction

The choice of microphone is perhaps the most critical stage in any vocal recording, but it is only the starting point. The acoustic signal, once converted to the electrical domain, must at some point return to the acoustic world via a loudspeaker. In the interim it will need to be boosted, attenuated, processed, mixed with other sources, and most importantly, stored permanently in some manner for later playback. What follows in this section is an overview of the most important aspects of the recording chain with a view to recording the voice—the microphone preamp stage; the mixer channel strip; the mixer outputs; the additional processing that might be required to correct or enhance the original recording; the storage medium for the acoustic signals. They will be also be considered in a general sense for although, by way of example, audio mixers vary in terms of individual design or configuration, they all share a common purpose. Also, with the exception of the microphone preamp, which must by necessity be based in the analog domain, all other components might be considered as analog hardware, digital hardware, or digital software. The music technology industry, as with wider IT, computing, and engineering disciplines, has seen the benefit of significant increases in computing power, memory, and storage, with ever falling costs. As such, it is pos-

sible for an entire "traditional" recording studio to exist on a modern laptop, running digital audio workstation software together with some associated front-end audio and MIDI interfacing hardware, often with three-figure track counts and software emulations of classic analog hardware, for a fraction of the price of the original. In such cases, the basic functionality of the digital software or hardware parallels that of the original analog hardware, and hence the terms used to describe them become interchangeable —and this is often because the digital implementation is designed to function, sound, and even look like the analog hardware it is supposed to emulate.

The Microphone Preamp Stage

The microphone preamp is where the electrical input signal is conditioned so that it is suitable for further processing as part of the recording chain. These later stages may be analog or digital (hardware or software) and in the latter examples, the preamp will actually condition the signal ready for sampling as a digital signal using an analog-to-digital converter. If the complete recording setup is computer or even laptop based, it may be that the only additional hardware required is an audio interface consisting of a number of channels of microphone preamps, additional line level inputs, and several audio outputs. This will then be connected to the computer via a standard hardware communications protocol such as USB, USB2, Firewire, or PCI/PCI Express. Whatever the application, the preamp controls will include most, if not all, of the components presented in the mixing desk overview in Figure 4–13 and described in the following.

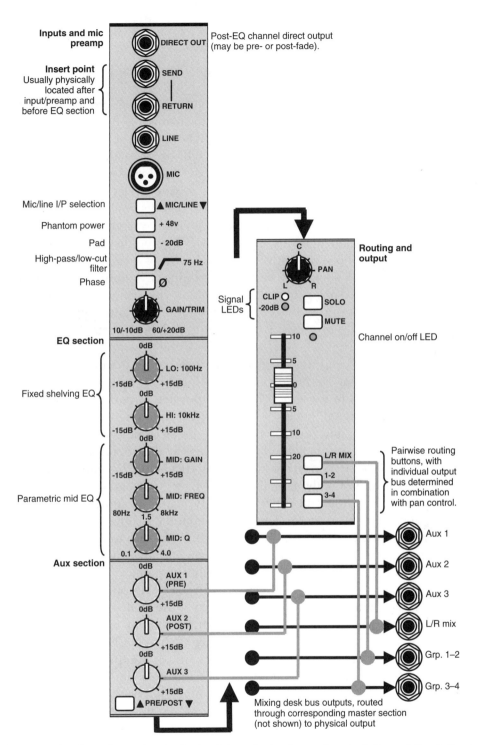

Figure 4–13. *Overview of a typical mixing desk channel, consisting of the following sections: (a) an input connection and microphone preamp stage; (b) EQ with two fixed band shelving controls and one parametric mid; (c) three aux sends, one pre-fade, one post-fade, and one selectable between the two; (d) routing and output to L/R mix bus and up to four additional groups. Any mixer design will consist of many such repeated channels, together with output buses and an appropriate overall master section.*

Mic/Line Input

Microphones have very low output levels—10 mV being a typical example—whereas analogue audio circuitry works with signals around 1 V. If the signal were any quieter it would be subject to the noise floor of the system itself, and therefore a microphone signal must typically be boosted about 100 times—equivalent to 40 dB of gain. In reality, the signal from the microphone depends on the level of the sound source. A very loud sound will not need any gain (0 dB) whereas a very quiet sound will need a considerable amount (up to 80 dB). Typical preamps will offer somewhere in the region of 60 dB of gain, and it is always worth remembering that the more gain that is applied, the more noise will be added to the source signal; hence, it is always worth selecting and positioning microphones to capture the best level of sound that is possible for a given recording environment. Additionally, as stated in the introduction under the Microphones section, condenser microphones will generally produce a higher level of signal output compared with a dynamic microphone and therefore require less gain and result in a lower noise floor. One of the skills of making good recordings is to optimize the gain levels at all stages of the recording chain—that is, to get the signal as high as possible, therefore minimizing noise, while at all times avoiding clipping distortion. In the section Other Important Microphone Considerations, the overload point of the microphone was considered in terms of the maximum displacement of the diaphragm. In this case the microphone preamp can also overload and cause clipping distortion if it is driven with a signal level from the microphone that is too high.

Note that there are many places on a typical mixing desk where a signal might be boosted so that clipping distortion will occur, with the preamp being only the first in the signal chain. As such, most mixing desks provide some form of LED based signal level meters to provide a visual warning as to the possibilities of clipping distortion. This may be in the form of a complex multisegment bar graph, or a simple single overload LED that will flash when the signal level is too high. The latter type of metering might well be located in the preamp stage. If the preamp is part of an audio interface, rather than a mixer, overload warning LEDs will also generally be incorporated as part of the preamp. The overload LED might also be multifunction—green to indicate a signal is present, perhaps at −20 dB, red to indicate a couple of dBs below the clipping point.

Mixer channels and audio interfaces are typically designed to be able to accommodate different types of audio signal. Whereas a microphone input can be very variable in nature and require significant gain, a *line level* input will have been preamplified at source, and is typically the analog audio signal that is produced by an electrically powered device such as a CD player, synthesizer keyboard, or computer soundcard output. Consumer audio equipment has a common reference of −10 dBV, with professional audio devices having a reference value of +4 dBu (note the change in dB reference!). As with microphones, the actual input level can vary, and hence gain—or attenuation—may need to be applied at the preamp input, although ideally the level will operate around these quoted figures. Most professional audio equipment can deal with consumer or professional levels, and it is worth checking that settings are appropriate for the connections being used, or distortion in the signal may result. The important thing to note here, however, is that microphone input levels are considerably lower than line level, and require appropriate interfacing and gain levels to work correctly with the analog input of the signal chain. A button marked as *mic/line, line,* or similarly might well be used to select between the microphone or line level input as the source for the signal path that follows. With preamps that also serve as audio interfaces for computer based systems, these options may be controlled via software, rather than using physical hardware in the forms of buttons or switches.

Input Connection

One of the clear differences between the two inputs is the nature of the connector. A line level input might be supplied using a quarter-inch jack, using mono (unbalanced) or stereo (balanced) connectors, a stereo 3/8" mini jack, or a phono type connector (usually found on domestic stereo equipment). Most microphone connections are supplied using what is known as an XLR connector—a three-pin design, with male/female connections. The female end will connect to the capsule of the microphone, with the male end connecting to the preamp input. The connectors are rugged, clicking into place at both ends to ensure a secure connection, and long cable lengths (up to 20 m) may be used as they are excellent at rejecting interference and noise. This is due to their *balanced* operation that carries the same audio signal along

two of the connecting pins, with one phase inverted with respect to the other.

Phantom Power

The balanced XLR microphone connector/cable design can also be used to carry a +48 V dc source suitable for powering a condenser microphone. A button or switch will be supplied for this purpose, usually per preamp input, but may be applied globally to all preamps from a single switch on lower-cost pream or mixer designs. It is important to always plug the microphone in first before switching the phantom power on or off, making sure that the gain controls/faders are down to avoid a characteristic thump that may cause damage to loudspeakers or to hearing if a sufficiently high level. Note that dynamic microphones or battery powered condensers should not be affected if they are supplied with phantom power by mistake or through limitations of preamp design. This voltage source is called "phantom" power because it is invisible to those microphones that do not use it due to the balanced nature of the connections—it will also not affect the actual audio signal. If the preamp itself is not capable of supplying phantom power (sometimes the case on portable recorders), either battery powered condenser microphones or an external phantom power supply will have to be used.

Trim/Gain

This (usually) rotary control is where a microphone signal can actually be boosted, or a line level signal boosted or attenuated (trimmed). The same control will be used for both options, usually with the range of cut/boost altered accordingly.

With some computer based systems, this gain might be controlled digitally, although note that this would be *digital* control of *analog* gain. Once converted to a sampled digital signal, it is not possible to increase gain levels further without losing signal information or resolution. Some computer controlled preamps will allow additional digital gain or attenuation to be applied once a signal has been converted to the digital domain, but this cannot compensate for low signal levels at the recording stage.

If using a computer based system, it is therefore important to check what options are available for control of signal levels. If there are actual rotary controls by each microphone preamp, this would indicate analog gain control, and additional gain stages in the signal path should not be used as they would be operating on the digital signal information. If there are no such controls, it is likely that the analog gain settings are controlled digitally. This can be very useful as it allows precise and accurate level setting, and these settings can then be saved for recall as part of a later session.

Pad

This is designed to automatically attenuate the microphone input signal level by a preset amount, typically in the order of 20 dB. This is not standard in all preamps, and indeed some microphones may have small switches built into the capsule to achieve the same result—in which case it is important to ensure that both are not selected! Such attenuation is useful for very high level signals to bring them back within the effective operational range of the preamp for situations when the trim/gain control is turned all the way down but signal clipping is still evident.

High-Pass/Low-Cut Filter

As with the pad control, the high-pass/low-cut filter is not always included as part of the preamp design and the button/switch may even be located elsewhere on the channel signal path. For instance, on analog mixing desks it is often found somewhere in the channel EQ section as it may be considered as a certain type of frequency specific gain (as are all forms of EQ), but it is really designed to condition the signal at the input stage rather than to manipulate it further at some later point. As with the pad control, it may also be incorporated as part of the microphone itself. It is designed to remove low frequency components (hence *low-cut*) from the input signal below a specific value given in Hz, while allowing the remainder of the signal above this value to pass through unchanged (hence *high-pass*). This value may be fixed at 75 or 100 Hz (or similar level), with some microphones giving a variety of options possibly up as far as 150 Hz. It can be used to compensate for undesirable proximity effect bass-boost, and can help to remove low frequency noise originating from mains hum (50/60 Hz), room modes (can be problematic below 300 Hz), or handling noise. It is good practice to make use of it when recording to avoid the capture of such problematic audio components, but knowledge relating to the spectral content of the acoustic source is important. For instance, the adult male voice has a typical fundamental frequency, f0, of 110 Hz, whereas with the female voice it is in the region of f0 = 170 Hz. With respect to the singing voice, a bass singer's lowest fundamental will be in the region of f0 = 65 Hz, for a tenor, f0 = 123 Hz, an alto, f0 = 175 Hz, and a soprano, f0 = 260 Hz. Hence, in most cases, careful use of a correctly set high-pass filter before or at the preamp stage can help to minimize low potential low frequency problems with no impact on the source material.

Phase

Again, this is not always found in all preamp designs, and it may be implemented in the digital domain rather than in analog hardware. The button inverts the phase of the signal, and when heard in isolation it will have no perceptual change on what is heard from the loudspeakers. However, it may be useful for incorrectly wired XLR cables and is particularly important when using many spaced microphones on an acoustic source, as the time of arrival differences between microphones may result in phase cancellation effects (see Chapter 5, section on Stereo Recording). The phase button allows this potentially undesirable effect to be checked and compensated for, by reversing the phase of one of the signals. It is also used when using mid-side stereo microphone techniques (see Chapter 5, Stereo Recording).

Conditioning the Signal Further—Inserts and EQ

Once beyond the microphone preamp, the audio signal is ready for additional processing, shaping, and conditioning. With a digital system the signal will now be operated on entirely in the digital domain, implying the quality and integrity of the signal should be maintained within the limitations of the algorithms used and the resolution of the digital information in terms of sample rate and bit depth. With an analog system, the signal will still be susceptible to additional noise and the quality and character of the underlying analog circuitry. In both cases, caution should be exercised, particularly when recording for the first time, and material should be carefully auditioned to ensure that quality and integrity of the source information is maintained.

Insert Point

On an analog mixing desk, generally the next component in the signal chain is an insert point, a physical audio input/output connection that makes a break in the signal flow path and hence allows additional audio processing devices to be inserted or "patched" into this chain. The most commonly used devices are compressors, noise gates, and high quality equalizers, and they will only work on the channel to which they are connected (an important distinction to make as will be considered later with auxiliary sends). With nothing connected to the insert point an internal switch is closed so that the signal continues unhindered. Insert points are generally not included on computer based audio interface/microphone preamps, mainly because this would require a further stage of digital-to-analog and analog-to-digital conversion, increasing costs, and possibly compromising quality. Digital hardware may offer limited insert options or none at all. Both such systems usually compensate for these shortcomings with included software algorithms that can be used in exactly the same manner as third party hardware, although generally not at the same perceived quality as their analog counterparts, and often with additional computer processing overheads that may make live recording work difficult. The solution here would be to use an external, stand-alone microphone preamp, followed by the desired external processing unit, which would in turn then be connected to the audio input. Note also that top of the line analog desks may also have built compressors and noise gates on every audio input channel instead of insert points.

The EQ Section

After the insert point come the equalization (EQ) controls. EQ is a process by which a specific part or parts of the audible frequency spectrum are either cut or boosted, in order to change the quality or timbre of the sound—it is essentially a frequency selective gain control. There are many different types of EQ common to recording use but all offer controls that allow the user to determine what frequency, or range of frequencies, should be adjusted, or alternatively what range of frequencies should be unchanged

(measured in Hz), and by how much this selection should be adjusted (gain, cut/boost, amplification/attenuation, measured in dB). These controls are defined as *center frequency* (or just frequency), *gain*, *Q*, and *bandwidth*, and are highlighted in the simplified frequency response graph shown in Figure 4–14.

The frequency about which the EQ control operates is the center frequency (in Hz). The amount of gain or, more commonly, cut or boost applied at this frequency is given in dB, and the range of frequencies over which this cut or boost is applied is determined by the bandwidth of the EQ control. Related to bandwidth is the Q—or quality factor— which describes the shape of the EQ response curve as the ratio of the center frequency to the difference between the upper and lower frequencies that are being affected. The upper and lower frequencies are defined to be the points at

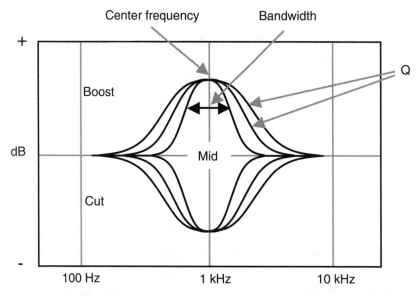

Figure 4–14. *A simplified frequency response demonstrating the effect EQ has on the spectrum of a signal and the terms used to describe the characteristics of the applied EQ.*

which the cut or boost in question is 3 dB less or more than that of the center frequency. Many EQ circuits are designed to be *constant Q*; that is, the shape of the response curve is designed to stay the same as the gain varies, maintaining a constant musical bandwidth that is more naturally pleasing and accurate sounding to our ears. Despite being called "constant Q" it is actually the Q value that changes, while the effective bandwidth of the circuit stays the same.

The higher the Q value, the narrower the range of frequencies being affected; the lower the Q value, the wider the range being affected. Practically speaking, one octave (Q = 1.5) is a good value to start out with for most general EQ tasks. An octave is generally narrow enough to get close to the frequencies required, yet wide enough not to color the sound too much. The main types of EQ are summarized as follows.

Fixed or Shelving EQ. These are EQ circuits fixed to work at a specific frequency, generally set such that high (treble) = 10 kHz and low (bass) = 100 Hz; they are designed to cut or boost the frequency content of the signal above or below this fixed point. With typical domestic analog audio systems the frequency response of bass and treble controls is usually very gradual and the tonal variation is very limited (Figure 4–15). On an analog mixing desk there is a much sharper cutoff point, resulting in a "shelf" effect on the frequency response graph; hence, they are often called *shelving EQ*. Low end desks and guitar amps will often add a third middle control, fixed somewhere around 2 kHz, with a fixed bandwidth of a couple of octaves or so. This will have a typical bell-shaped frequency response curve as pre-

sented in Figure 4–14. The frequency response for three bands of fixed EQ, effectively giving bass, middle, and treble controls, is shown in Figure 4–15.

Semiparametric EQ or "Swept Mid." With this type of EQ the bandwidth is still fixed but the center frequency is adjustable so that a specific frequency can be "dialed in." Two controls are therefore provided, center frequency and gain. The best way to use these controls is to turn the boost all the way up and sweep through the range of frequencies, listening for where the sound peaks or stands out too much due to a particular resonance. Then adjust to suit.

Parametric EQ. This is the same as the semiparametric EQ but now has an extra control added to allow the Q to be changed. Generally if a studio has outboard EQ it will consist of multiband parametric EQs that can be added to the signal path via the insert point to augment or replace the desk EQ.

Graphic EQ. This is the type of EQ that is familiar to most people and is the easiest and most intuitive to operate. It has fixed bandwidth and center frequencies, but instead of having two or three rotary controls it will have a number (usually 10 or more) of sliders spaced evenly across the frequency spectrum. The center frequencies for a 10-band graphic EQ are: 31 Hz, 63 Hz, 125 Hz, 250 Hz, 500 Hz, 1 kHz, 2 kHz, 4 kHz, 8kHz, and 16 kHz. And for a 30-band EQ the frequencies are: 25 Hz, 31 Hz, 40 Hz, 50 Hz, 63 Hz, 80 Hz . . . 10 kHz, 12.5 kHz, 16 kHz, 20 kHz.

The range of cut/boost is usually 12 dB, although some allow greater adjustment. Looking at the slider positions gives a good indication of what the

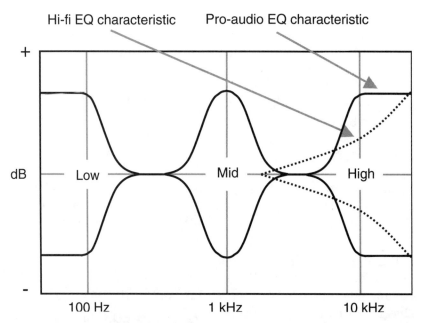

Hi-fi EQ characteristic   Pro-audio EQ characteristic

Figure 4–15. *A simplified frequency response demonstrating three fixed bands of EQ, high and low shelving at 10 kHz and 100 Hz, respectively, and a single band of middle EQ at 1 kHz. Also shown is an example of how the EQ characteristics of a "hi-fi" treble control differs from that of a similar pro-audio EQ as found on most mixing desks.*

resulting frequency response curve looks like. The bandwidth of each slider depends upon its number. As a graphic EQ is designed to cover the whole frequency spectrum, 10 sliders implies that each is one octave wide. The most common example is a 31-band, 1/3-octave bandwidth, graphic EQ and it is used extensively when sound engineering for live performance (see Operational Guidelines below), although they have less application and are therefore less common in the recording studio.

Paragraphic EQ. This is a digital version of an analog EQ circuit and is exactly the same as a standard parametric EQ, except this implementation allows the frequency response curve of the EQ settings to be visualized on a screen and it

is usually possible to interact directly with the graphics. The additional advantage of a digital implementation is that center frequencies can now operate over the entire audible spectrum and accurate setting, editing, and recall of the controls is possible. However, most digital or software implementations usually default by giving the user the traditional analog set-up of high and low fixed band shelving EQ combined with two fully parametric mid-range bands.

Notch Filter. A specific form of EQ with a very narrow bandwidth, this is designed to eliminate problem frequencies. An example would be using a series of notch filters to remove 50/60 Hz mains hum and its associated harmonic frequencies.

Note that with most analog mixing desk, the whole EQ section can be bypassed from a single button. This is useful for doing A/B comparisons, or minimizing the possibility of noise being added to a recording. If EQ is not required when recording, the EQ section should be in bypass mode, and this also avoids the problem of accidentally making a recording with the EQ of a previous session being applied to the channel signal path being used. In addition to basic fixed band bass and treble shelving EQ, a good analog desk will usually offer two bands of swept mid, ranging from low to high frequency with overlaps between low and low-mid, low-mid and high-mid, and high-mid and high bands. In this way the entire audible frequency range is covered sufficiently, and one or both of these mid-band controls may additionally offer full parametric control. The low-cut/high-pass filter may also be found with these controls as discussed in the section The Microphone Preamp Stage.

Interfacing with External Devices—The Auxiliary Section

One method of connecting external equipment to the input signal path has already been discussed in the form of the post-preamp insert point that provides a physical break along this line of communication. The other method for connecting additional audio processing devices is via the *auxiliary send* controls. These are essentially additional outputs —also known as *buses*—from the desk sourced from each input channel. In this way one physical audio output can carry a signal sourced from every audio input, allowing considerable routing flexibility.

The auxiliary (aux) sends are usually the next physical set of controls along the signal chain, and although they might not be accommodated physically in digital audio interfacing hardware, the accompanying digital audio software will allow similar routing to be configured internally (or externally to general, rather than specific aux send, hardware audio outputs). As most such software is based on analog mixing desk design, these internal auxiliary sends operate in the same manner as their analog counterparts and are described similarly, and so what follows again applies directly to analog/digital hardware or software implementations.

Each aux send works like a separate mixer level control and is independent of any main mix settings controlled, for instance, by the main channel faders. Hence, a mixer with a main stereo output and four aux sends per channel could potentially provide five completely different mixes of the same sound input sources. There are two main uses for auxiliary sends, described as follows.

Foldback

If a vocalist is being recorded in an acoustically isolated studio room or vocal booth, she will want to hear herself, any backing tracks that have already recorded, and potentially any other performers, over her headphones. An auxiliary send can supply an appropriate signal to the headphones for this. If there is more than one singer or musician, each requiring a separate mix, then each individual foldback mix is controlled by its own aux send. Once the vocalist is happy with her headphone mix it is important not to change it. If the level of the vocal source has to be adjusted mid-take, perhaps because there is danger of clipping, this could also alter the foldback headphone mix. For this reason, aux sends used for foldback must be set as *pre-fade*—they are not affected by the channel fader setting, allowing a complete submix to be established that is independent of what the studio engineer will be hearing.

Effects

The other major use for the aux sends is to send a submix of the input signals to an effects unit for additional processing. The most common of these is reverb. Note that reverb and related digital effects are different from how compressors, gates, and to an extent EQs work. These latter devices are designed to operate on and alter the characteristics of an individual audio signal and can behave in a very nonlinear manner. Nonlinear in this case means that the output from two summed input signals, passed through the device, is not equivalent to each being processed separately, passed through separate devices (with the same settings) and then summed. Reverb and delay based effects are linear devices, and so one effect unit can be used with an input derived from many individual summed sources, and the result is equivalent to each individual component being processed by its own

reverb device, as shown in Figure 4–16. In terms of how the aux sends are used in this context, during mixing a separate balance of signals will be sent to the reverb unit using one (or two if in stereo) aux send controls. In this case the level arriving at the reverb input from each channel *should* be controlled by the fader. If a channel is faded down the reverb should fade also. This is therefore done using a *post-fade* auxiliary. Note that this implies that there are two places on the signal path where the actual level of the aux send is determined—the aux send level control and the gain/fader control itself.

Depending on the design of the mixing desk and the budget available, there will be at least one auxiliary send per channel, typically running up to as many as eight (or more). Some of these controls may be fixed as pre- or post-fade, with others being switchable between pre- and post-fade operation, often for economical reasons. Similarly, some mixing desks offer a reduced set of hardware controls with the option to select which aux send bus (for instance aux send 5 or aux send 7) is associated with a particular physical aux send level control, saving on both size and circuitry and hence being more economical to manufacture.

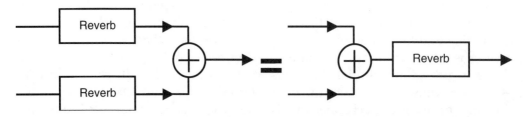

Figure 4–16. *Reverb and other similar delay based effects are linear devices. This means that one effect unit can be used with an input derived from many individual summed sources, and the result is equivalent to each individual component being processed by its own reverb device.*

Routing and Output

So far the signal has arrived at the pre-amp and either been conditioned for further processing (and possibly processed using input channel EQ or third party devices) or converted to a sampled signal ready for similar treatment in the digital domain. It is possible that an effective submix or copy of the signal has been routed via the auxiliary sends to provide foldback for the performer or further effects processing options, but so far it has not been considered where the signal should go in terms of listening to the signal from the engineer's point of view, or where it should be routed to for actual recording and storage. And, hardware or software devices, mixing desks, or audio interfaces. All are designed to offer significant flexibility in terms of signal routing, and hence a signal does not usually default to an output—this has to be actively decided upon and acted on. This takes place in the routing/output section of the signal flow path.

Routing

A series of buttons are used to send the signal from the channel to one of the audio outputs—either directly to the main *left/right mix bus* or to an additional output, usually called a group output, that could, for instance, be connected (either physically or virtually) to an audio track for recording. These buttons usually assign the audio input equally to a pair of buses—left and right; 1 and 2, etc.

Pan (Panoramic Potentiometer)

This is a rotary control (sometimes implemented as a horizontal slider in software) that is used to position the audio signal within the stereo field (between left and right stereo loud-speaker and hence left or right mix bus) or is alternatively used to direct a signal between odd/even buses or group outputs. For instance, pressing the routing button associated with buses 1 and 2, with the pan control in the center position, will send the same signal to these same two outputs. Moving the pan control so that it is hard left will send the signal to output bus 1 only. Moving it to the extreme right will send the signal to output 2 only. Similarly, if the main left/right mix routing button is pressed, with the pan control centre, the signal will be heard coming equally from both loudspeakers (assuming they are connected correctly and the master section is operating as it should—see below!). Panning slowly hard left will result in the stereo image of the signal seeming to move to the left until it is heard in the left-hand speaker only. Now panning slowly from hard left through the center position to hard right will shift the stereo image from the left-hand speaker, through the center point between the two speakers (where it is reproduced with equal level from both speakers) until it is heard only in the right-hand speaker. Stereo imaging, recording, and reproduction will be discussed further in Chapter 5, Stereo Recording.

Fader

This is usually the only control that operates in a straight and vertical line! It is used to alter the level of the input signal as it leaves the channel. The long vertical nature of the fader facilitates ease of use and enables better mixing, while providing an at–a-glance reference to what each of the input channels is doing. The fader adjusts the level of the channel signal between minus infinity dB (no fader can reduce the signal completely to nothing as this is a logarithmic scale, and hence *tends* to zero although will never actually reach it; however, it can be assumed that the result is essentially absolute silence) and, for instance, +10 dB. Hence, it is actually possible to also boost the signal, rather than just attenuate it (although not as much as with the preamp gain control). Normal operating position is at the unity gain, 0 dB mark—so that the channel fader neither attenuates nor boosts the signal over and above the setting of the preamp gain control.

In addition the routing/output section may have a *solo* button to quickly isolate the signal for auditioning without any additional accompaniment. It may also have a *mute* or *on/off* button to disable the channel.

Finally, with respect to the signal inputs, if the input preamps are based around a mixing desk rather than an audio interface, some provision will be made for inputs from a multitrack—this may be analog or digital hardware, or multiple audio outputs from a computer based system. Depending on the size and configuration of the desk, these may connect to the line inputs of spare input channels. However, it is most common to make use of the circuitry available on the same input channel, and so the preamp/input stage will also have a physical *tape input* or *tape return input* (it may also have a *direct out* for sending directly to the multitrack), and at the very least an additional rotary level and pan control at some point along the signal path to control this additional input signal. In such a design—called an *inline* design (as opposed to a *split* design where the tape inputs have their own dedicated channels)—it is also common to have buttons that switch some of the aux

sends, or some of the EQ section, from the input path to the tape return path. Finally, once recording has been completed it is possible to swap the signal paths around—the physical inputs become associated with the tape return path, and the signals from the multitrack can then be mixed and controlled via the full features offered by the main input channel. Although very flexible, this can also be a source of considerable confusion, and so it is important to refer to the manual of the particular mixer being used. Note that with a software system, this arrangement is less common as there is a one-to-one relationship between audio tracks (containing recorded audio signals) and audio channels (where these signals are conditioned, mixed, and processed). Flexibility here is offered in terms of how audio hardware inputs and outputs are routed appropriately to each audio track. Typically in the hardware world there are more input channels on the mixing desk than there are tape tracks to record to or audio inputs to connect to.

Hearing the Result—The Group Outputs and Master Section

Once the microphone input has had its gain optimized and further conditioned via EQ, insert effects, post-fade auxiliary send effects and submixed to the performer via pre-fade aux sends routed to an appropriate output bus, there is still every chance that nothing will be heard! So far the signal path has dealt with an input signal; this signal must be sent to an appropriate physical output section of the desk or audio interface, and the outputs all have their own individual settings and controls.

Groups and Subgroups

In general the term *group* is used when the signal is sent to a physical audio output and *subgroup* is used to send the signal somewhere else within the signal architecture—usually to the output section. In this way a whole number of individual signals, such as an individually close-miked choir, might be recorded to one mono or two stereo tracks by routing them to a group first. Alternatively, when mixing, these many tracks might be altered in unison, thus reducing the number of fingers required to adjust the level of the whole ensemble by sending them to a subgroup first. In reality the same set of physical faders will be used for both tasks; in the latter case the signals will be further routed to the main left/right outputs. In the first, more recording focused example, they will be sent directly out to an audio track input. Groups are therefore very simple and will typically consist of a left/right (L/R) mix routing button to send the signal on further to the main L/R outputs, a pan control (for odd/even group assignment), solo, mute, possibly an assign mono button (sends signals equally to L/R bus, or odd/even physical outputs), and finally a fader. In software implementations, groups are really only used to simplify the mixing process, or to route to actual physical audio outputs, rather than to submix to a track. However, generally the routing options provided are very flexible and so they can be used in any way the operator sees fit to condition, route, and mix input signals and audio tracks.

The Master Fader

This controls the main L/R mix bus output, and hence generally what is sent to the stereo loudspeakers and any stereo recording devices (such as a DAT recorder). The maximum value is usually 0 dB, so it can only be used to attenuate the overall mix rather than boost it further (compare with the channel faders as discussed above).

The Auxiliary Masters

Each channel auxiliary send will have a master level control, generally a rotary control perhaps with a solo button and some additional routing options (for instance, to the headphone outputs for creating performer foldback mixes). Note now that for a post-fade aux send there are three places where the signal level might be controlled: the input channel aux send, the main input fader (plus of course the associated input gain control), and now the auxiliary master. In a software implementation the auxiliary master is often associated directly with an input level control on the software effect itself.

Effects Returns

Often found in stereo pairs, these very simple input channels are usually used to add the signal returning from the aux send effects units to the main mix—for instance, the original signal now with added reverb. They will have a level control, and a balance control (to balance the left/right signals, as panning is not strictly appropriate for a stereo signal), and routing options to allow pairwise assignment to the groups, main L/R output (for effects for the overall mix), or headphones (to send an effected signal to the foldback mix). The effects returns may also be used as simple, general stereo input channels for stereo sources such as keyboards or CD players. They may also appear in hardware as a small subset of the control surface with rotary level controls, or as specific, full length stereo input channels. In software the latter will always apply.

Finally, in the master section there will be a number of options to select what you are actually listening to via the main loudspeakers (also called monitors), and via any special headphone outputs. Possible options include the (obvious) main L/R mix bus, the sum of the tape returns, pairs of pre-fade auxiliary sends (to check foldback or send foldback to the performers), post-fade auxiliary sends (to listen to effects submixes), external inputs (perhaps from a specific two-track stereo input using phono connectors), or a mono version of the stereo mix to check to see how it sounds in mono, or to remove problems of using only one signal to feed stereo headphones (otherwise the performer would hear the result in one ear only and this can be off-putting). With a software mixer, there will be similar options, but in this case it allows the user to select to what physical audio outputs the signals must be sent. Note also that in both hardware and software it is usual for groups and master outputs to have insert points to add specific effects (such as stereo compression or EQ) to the whole mix.

Talkback

Hardware systems will also generally provide a simple means of communicating with the performers in a separate recording space via a small microphone placed near the surface of the mixing desk itself. This is called a talkback mike and is operated via a specific microphone. The signal is usually routed to either the pre-fade auxiliaries, headphones, or both. It might also be possible to route the signal to a group output, allowing the studio engineer to dictate notes directly to an audio track before or after recording. When talkback is engaged, to prevent feedback and allow the engineer to hear the performers, the control room outputs will usually be automatically attenuated by a preset amount.

Insert Effects

Insert effects, as already introduced in the section Conditioning the Signal Further—Inserts and EQ, are generally nonlinear processes designed to operate on the signal passed through them according to their specific spectral or time-varying characteristics. EQ is a very common example and has already been discussed in some length in this same chapter. Probably the two next most commonly used insert effects, which have a particular use when recording vocals, are *compressors* and *noise gates* (or just *gates*), both of which will be introduced in this section.

Dynamics and Compression

An audio compressor (and note that in this context compression refers to the process applied to an audio signal to alter its dynamic content, rather than the data compression that might be applied to an audio signal to store it in a more compact form as used in MP3 and similar formats) is designed to alter the dynamic nature of the audio track it is operating on. Put simply, "dynamics" refers to how the amplitude of a signal varies over time, with particularly *dynamic* material having some considerable variability in its overall amplitude. This might therefore refer to the difference between the loudest and softest parts of a piece of music, or the difference between the transient peaks and steady state aspects of an audio signal, both of which might manifest themselves in differences between the highest and lowest peaks in the audio waveform representation of the signal.

In the example presented in Figure 4–17, the pop music example has a clear difference between loudest and quietest parts of the mix. There are also clear transients that stand out from the steady state background level of the track. This is therefore an example of dynamics in the recording. By way of contrast, the rock music track is clearly less dynamic —transients are harder to make out, and there is no real difference between the loudest peaks and the rest of the track. The overall average level of the rock track is greater than that of the pop music example (indicated by the denser waveform), although the maximum peak level in both is actually the same. The result is that we perceive the rock track as being loud.

Hence, a compressor is used to automatically alter the dynamic content of an audio signal passed through it by leaving the quieter aspects of the signal untouched, and reducing the amplitude of the louder sections. As a result, the difference between the loudest and quietest parts is decreased and so the dynamics of the signal are reduced. Additionally, by reducing the peaks in the signal, the overall track can be boosted in gain, and so the track is made to appear louder. This is the basic operation of any compressor—it reduces the level of the loudest parts of a signal, and by doing so makes it possible to boost the overall level of the quieter sections (without introducing clipping or distortion), ultimately reducing the overall dynamic content.

Setting Up and Using a Compressor or Dynamics Processor

The most important consideration when using a compressor or more general dynamics processor is that it is almost always connected as an *insert* effect— not via an auxiliary bus—as it should process the whole signal present in a particular channel. A typical device will consist of a number of rotary controls that work in a very interactive manner; that is, the setting for one will have an influence on how the others operate. This feature, together with the fact that

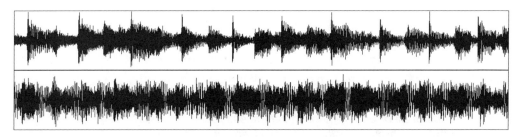

Figure 4–17. *Dynamics and loudness in music. The upper track is a 5-second example from a pop song where there is a clear difference between the loudest and quietest aspects of the audio. The lower example is a 5-second extract from a rock track. The difference between loudest and quietest aspects of the signal is less obvious.*

the compression effect is sometimes difficult to perceive (it is not obvious or dramatic like other common effects such as reverb or EQ), can lead to confusion in terms of how the device works and how it alters the audio signal, and so some care, a good understanding of the underlying principles, and careful listening are required.

The basic functional operation of a compressor is shown in Figure 4–18, where it is clear that the audio input is passed through to the output via a *voltage controlled amplifier* (VCA), represented here by a circle with a cross within it, showing that the value of the signal level is going to be multiplied by some factor at this point. Note also that before this happens the signal is tapped off the main input-output path, into what is called the *side-chain*. There are two operations that occur here; the first is that the signal level is monitored, and the second is that based on the result

of this monitoring process, the gain control of the VCA is altered. The signal level is monitored to check whether it exceeds a user-defined *threshold,* and all such dynamics processors work on this threshold principle; hence, this is the first control to be considered.

Threshold. This determines the level at which the side-chain level detector will act on the VCA and hence where the compression begins. Consider the example presented in Figure 4–19. If the sound level at the input is below the threshold (set here at –10 dB), nothing happens as shown in Figure 4–19(a). Once the signal is greater than the threshold (or alternatively, if the threshold control is reduced further), the compressor starts working, automatically reducing the output gain (Figure 4–19[c]), by a predetermined amount (Figure 4–19[b]).

Tip: –10 dB is a good value to start with for very subtle compression, and

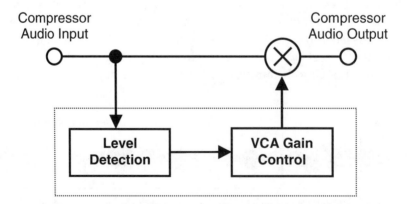

Figure 4–18. *The functional block diagram representation of a compressor or other typical dynamics processor. The input signal passes through to the output via an amplifier where the signal level can be controlled. The signal is also monitored in parallel to this in the side-chain. The value of the signal level in the side-chain determines how much (if any) gain or attenuation is applied at the amplifier in the input/output path.*

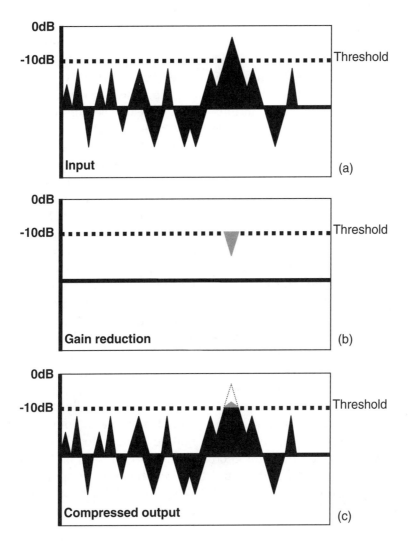

Figure 4–19. *The operation of a compressor is determined by setting a threshold value. (a) As long as the input signal is below the threshold value nothing happens. (b) When the input signal exceeds the threshold, gain reduction will be applied according to the settings of the ratio control. (c) The result is that the output signal will have had the peak that exceeded the threshold value reduced in level (compressed).*

–20 dB better for something a bit more noticeable.

Ratio. The amount of gain reduction applied is set using the ratio control. This refers to how much the signal level will be reduced by—how the detector will act on the VCA gain control. A ratio of 1:1 will do nothing. A ratio of 2:1 means that the signal crossing the threshold will have its level reduced by a factor of two. Alternatively, for every

2 dB over the threshold level, the output will only rise by 1 dB. A ratio of 4:1 means that these peaks will have their level reduced by a factor of four: for every 4 dB over the threshold there will only be 1 dB rise in the output. An infinite ratio (often referred to as *limiting*) tells the compressor to never let the input signal get higher than the threshold.

Tip: A ratio of 3:1 is a good starting point, enough to make a difference to significant peaks but not to the detriment of the overall signal quality. Note also that the threshold and ratio controls are very much linked. Reducing the threshold or increasing the ratio will result in a very similar effect—the output is "more" compressed. In the former case this is because more of the signal is above the threshold level. In the latter example it is because more gain reduction is being applied. It is best to use the threshold control to vary the amount of compression applied and the ratio control to alter the sound quality of the result. The values given here are good starting points for voice recording and processing but experimentation and careful listening are the key!

Attack. Refers to the length of time after the threshold has first been crossed before the VCA is actually activated to reduce the level. Setting a higher attack value lets more of the peak transients through before attenuation begins.

Release. Once the signal has fallen back below the threshold, the release control determines the length of time before the compressor allows the signal level to return to normal. It sets how quickly the VCA "lets go" of the level control and allows the level to return to unity gain.

As the attack knob alters the start of a sound, the release control affects the end, making sounds sustain for a long time or cut off sharply.

Tip: The attack and release controls should really be considered for confident or advanced users, and can be used to make big changes to the dynamics of a signal. They can be used to accentuate transients in a signal, or remove them altogether. For vocal work, if available, use the *auto* mode switch that alters the attack and release automatically according to the signal content. If this is not available, a fast attack (15 ms) and a release value of 0.5 s are a good starting point for your own settings. If the release value is too short the result is the characteristic "pumping" sound of the compressor function turning on and off quickly. This is often heard on poorly set-up vocal microphones used to amplify spoken word over a public address system or on some radio broadcasts. If the release time is too long the signal is always compressed and gain reduction will continue to be applied even if the signal drops back below the threshold— the compressor never resets ready for the next signal peak.

Makeup Gain/Output. This is the post-compressor gain. As the act of compression reduces the overall level of signal peaks, the makeup gain boosts the level of the overall signal, effectively amplifying the quieter aspects of the signal, smoothing out the overall volume and giving a more consistent, but less dynamic, sound.

Tip: Always start with the output level control at 0 dB and then adjust to suit according to the amount of gain reduction being applied.

Metering. The LED metering on a compressor is the key to understanding what is actually going on when in use and consists of two multisegment displays. The left-hand meter displays the amount of *gain reduction* applied, increasing from right to left, with more LEDs lit implying more applied attenuation. Hence, by looking at the gain reduction meter and the behavior of the LEDs, it is possible to see by how much the signal is being compressed. It also gives feedback on the attack and release settings—the quicker the LEDs light up (also the more of them that are lit up), the faster the attack; the slower they take to return to 0 dB, the longer the release. The right-hand LED meter displays the *output level*, in this case operating from left to right. As such it can be used to compare the relative levels of the compressed and uncompressed signal by looking at this meter and using the b*ypass* switch. This last control turns the compressor function on or off—in bypass mode the audio signal passes through the device unaffected by any of the control settings.

Tip: The higher the ratio or the lower the threshold, the more gain reduction. For basic level control or subtle compression, no more than 6 dB of attenuation should be evidenced on the gain reduction LED meter.

Other Dynamics Processes— Gating

In addition to compression, there are other dynamics processes that might be applied as an insert effect, such as limiting, expansion, and compounding, although they may have less direct application to vocal recording and enhancement. However, one of the other commonly encountered devices that might be useful in some applications is a *gate*, essentially being a reverse compressor. Rather than attenuating loud signals, the gate attenuates only the quieter signals. It is often called a *noise gate* because it is usually used to eliminate noise when the desired signal is not present. It works on the same principle as a compressor, as shown in Figure 4–18, and so its operation is similarly determined by a threshold value/control as shown in Figure 4–20. Whereas a compressor attenuates a signal above the threshold value, a gate attenuates the signal below this value. If the input signal, Figure 4–20(a), is not high enough the gate is shut and nothing is heard at the output. When the signal exceeds the threshold value, the gate opens, Figure 4–20(b), allowing the signal to pass through for as long as the signal is greater than the threshold, Figure 4–20(c). A dedicated gate may have as many controls as a compressor, including ratio, attack, and release options, but is often included in its simplest form (a single threshold control) as part of a modern compressor or general dynamics processor. They are useful for cleaning up a voice signal if there is lots of background noise, but they have to be used with care as they can cut off the beginning or end of a word or phrase if it falls below the threshold, or quieter sections of a performance.

Aux Send Effects

By far the most commonly used studio effect, for voice or instrumental work, is reverberation. The development of close-miking techniques in popular music recording means that there is usually little of the recording room's acoustic

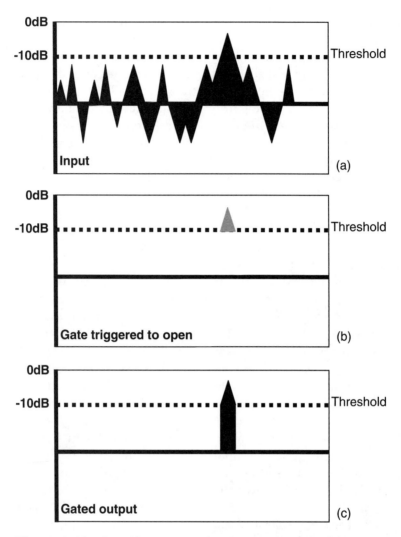

Figure 4–20. *As with a compressor, the operation of a gate is determined by setting a threshold value. (a) If the input signal is below the threshold value the gate will remain closed. (b) When the input signal exceeds the threshold, the gate will open for the duration for which the threshold value is exceeded. (c) The result is that the output signal will have low level signals removed (gated) and only consist of the louder sections.*

characteristics in the finished result. This is often unnatural and difficult to listen to and so artificial reverberation has to be added. This *reverberation*—or just *reverb*—gives a solid foundation for a recording by providing (usually) a uni-form acoustic context or "space" for the solo instrument or individual components of a more complex mix to exist, mirroring our perception of how real sounds behave in real acoustic spaces. Reverb also helps to impart a sense of distance. The more reverberant or effected sound there is compared with the direct or dry sound, the further back it is being pushed in the artificial reverberant space, the less clear it becomes and the more it occupies the background of a mix rather than the foreground.

Reverb belongs to the more general family of *delay* or *time based effects,* often called *digital effects* or *multi-effects,* and as they are linear processing devices (as discussed in the section Interfacing with External Devices—The Auxiliary Section), they all are designed to be connected to the mixing desk via the auxiliary sends, rather than the channel inserts.

Setting Up a Reverb or Delay Based Effects Unit

Once loaded up (if working in software) or turned on (in hardware), the mix or wet/dry control on the reverb/delay unit should always be set to 100% wet or 100% reverb. The auxiliary master controls and the stereo return controls should all be set to 0 dB by default and the amount of reverb/delay added to each channel signal can now be varied by turning up the appropriate individual channel aux send control. Hence, the balance of reverberated (wet) and unreverberated signals (dry) is controlled using the mixing desk itself. The main channel fader controls the dry signal, with the channel auxiliary send determining how much of this signal is sent to the reverb unit to become wet, and the stereo effect returns controlling the overall level of the reverb balanced against the channel dry signals. In general, overall reverb send/return levels of about 0 dB are optimal. However, it is possible to adjust the overall amount of reverberation and the balance of wet/dry sound to suit using the effects return level con-

trols in conjunction with the individual channel aux sends and main level faders. Note also that there may well be input and output level controls on the effects device itself and these should be set as high as possible, while ensuring at all times that there is no clipping or overload distortion—listen for any such detrimental effects and make use of any warning LEDs or visual feedback on the device that might indicate that distortion is occurring.

Reverb Parameters

Pre-Delay. On a reverb unit this is equivalent to changing the distance between the source and listener in a room; it adds a small delay between the direct, dry sound and the start of the reverb effect. Pre-delay therefore adds "space" to the overall reverb sound and stops the result from becoming too cluttered and "mushy" due to wet and dry signals becoming mixed immediately.

Reverb Type (or Preset). There are a number of different types of reverb type, depending on the size and type of space simulated, and these are named in an intuitive manner: e.g., big, medium, small, concert hall, room, warm (reverb is EQed to have more bass frequency energy relative to the treble content), bright (reverb is EQed to have more treble frequency energy relative to bass end content), etc. There are some other common types that need some additional explanation:

- **Plate reverb:** The very bright sound of an electro-mechanical plate reverb unit, commonly used in the 60s and 70s, and often used for vocals.
- **Reverse reverb:** A reverb effect that fades in and builds up rather than the usual fade out and decay.

- **Gated reverb:** The reverb is cut off quickly before it has a chance to decay using a built-in gate (see Insert Effects section); very dramatic when used on drums and characteristic of many of the drum tracks on songs recorded in the 80s.
- **Early reflections:** A more subtle effect than reverb, where an ambience is produced by modeling the first few sound reflections from the walls of a room, rather than the dense decaying reverberant tail; gives a natural sense of acoustic space without cluttering up or confusing the overall sound.

Reverb time. The time taken for the reverberation to decay to a certain level, usually defined as RT_{60} (see Chapter 3, section Sound Modification by a Space). This is an important parameter as it determines the total amount of reverb that will be added and helps to characterize the space being simulated. However, it will also act with the input and output level controls. A large space will generally have a long reverb time, but this will not be so evident if either the input level is low, or the wet/dry balance favors the original unreverberated signal, so as with compression, the results should be listened to carefully and levels set correctly for best results.

The Recording Medium

If a permanent record of a performance is required, then at some point the signal must be routed out from the mixing desk to some form of recording device. The recording device inputs will typically be connected to the main L/R mix outputs, the group outputs, or sometimes the channel *direct outs*. These last outputs are used to route a signal out of each individual channel, after the preamp stage, and as there is no possibility of further routing, processing, or conditioning, they are called *direct* outs. The recording medium/device itself can be characterized as follows.

Analog

This refers generally to the use of magnetic tape as the recording medium, consisting of a length of plastic material that is given a surface coating capable of retaining magnetic flux. When sound is recorded the tape is magnetized with a pattern of flux that is analogous to the acoustic signal itself. The record head that is used is basically an electromagnet with a small gap in it across which the tape passes. A playback head is used to read the magnetic signal and convert it back into the electrical domain. Common analog recorders use tape cassettes, reel-to-reel tape, or microcassettes (as found on voice recorders and answering machines). The signal is subject to additional noise due to the properties of the medium itself, leading to the requirement for, and development of, noise reduction techniques. This also means that the audio quality of second and higher generation copies of a master recording will deteriorate due to the accumulation of noise added with each subsequent copy made. The quality of the recording is also determined by how fast the tape is traveling over the record head and the width of the tape itself. They are much less common now than even 10 years ago due to the quality and affordability of modern digital recorders and as such should not really be considered for even basic vocal recording work. High-end analog machines are still used in the recording industry as they are perceived as having a better quality sound than many digital systems, even though they may be less accurate in terms of what they capture.

Digital

This refers to the storage of the original acoustic/electrical signal as a binary numerical representation consisting of 0s and 1s only. An analog electrical signal is converted to a digital representation via an analog-to-digital converter (ADC). The analog signal is divided into many individual static snapshots, and each snapshot is attributed a number according to the signal level. The number of snapshots taken per second is called the *sample rate* of the system. A digital compact disc uses a sample rate of 44.1 kHz; that is, the original signal is sampled 44,100 times per second. Other common sample rates found in the audio industry are 48 kHz (DAT, DVD) and 96 kHz (DVD-audio, HD-DVD). The higher the sample rate, then generally the better the quality of the recording or playback.

The number value attributed to each sample is determined by the number of bits, or *bit resolution*, of the system. CD is a 16-bit system, which means that each sample is represented by a 16-bit binary number—a series of 16 1s or 0s. This gives a total of $2^{16} = 65,536$ possible number values (or *quantization levels*) for each sample and determines the dynamic range of the system. With an analog system the dynamic range is determined by the difference between the loudest signal that can be carried/stored without distorting and the quietest signal above the noise floor inherent in any such device. With a digital system the dynamic range is determined by the number of bits the system can use to represent the digital

version of the signal. A 16-bit system has a dynamic range of about 96 dB. A 24-bit system has a theoretical dynamic range of 144 dB, although limitations in other aspects of the signal chain make this more likely to be of the order of 110 dB. DVD can accommodate 24-bit audio, as can DVD-audio and HD-DVD. The higher the bit resolution, the greater the dynamic range available and therefore, generally, the better quality the recording. There are a few points to note here, however. First, as with analog systems, signal levels need to be as high as possible; otherwise, a 24-bit ADC will use many fewer of its available bits to represent the signal, leading to a potential source of errors. Unlike analog systems, where pushing the level a little too high can give a desirable perceptual result without causing unwanted distortion, if the signal level exceeds the dynamic range of the ADC or digital medium, digital clipping will occur, which is a very undesirable effect. However, it is easily possible to make like-for-like copies without loss or degradation—all that is being physically copied is a series of numbers represented as 1s or 0s rather than a true analog of the signal that will be subject to the limitations of the medium itself. Finally, although it seems that higher sample rates and higher bit resolutions imply better quality audio, they also need more storage (as there are more numbers that need to be stored) and can put a strain on some recording systems unless they are optimized for high resolution digital recording. Wherever possible, opt for a 24-bit recording system. In terms of sample rate, it is often advisable to use a setting that matches the default value of the medium for which final delivery is intended. Therefore, if recording for CD, use a sample rate of 44.1 kHz at the recording stage and for DVD use 48 kHz. If a high sample rate is required or desired, again follow the guidelines of the delivery medium, with, for instance, 96 kHz for HD-DVD. For DVD, the appropriate high sample rate would also be 96 kHz, and a sample rate conversion to 48 kHz would be required prior to final mastering. As 96 kHz is an integer multiple of 48 kHz, this process is easy to compute while maintaining audio quality. Similarly, a high sample rate of 88.2 kHz is appropriate for a final 44.1 kHz CD release.

A digital-to-audio converter (DAC) performs the reverse task of taking this numerical representation of a sound and turning it back into an electric signal that can in turn be converted back to the acoustic domain. Although the stored data is digital, the actual media used takes many forms, including tapes (digital audio tape—DAT), video cassettes (ADAT—a digital multitrack format), CD-R (an optical medium), minidisk, computer hard disks, flash memory—in fact, pretty much any modern type of computer based storage device.

Two-Track (Stereo)

This is capable of recording (and playing back) two independent audio tracks. The most common application is for the medium to hold the final two-track mix (or master) for playback over a standard stereo audio system, although two independent mono tracks might also be possible. Hence, a two-track device is usually connected to the main L/R mix bus outputs. Typical examples include cassette, DAT, CD/CD-R, minidisk.

Multitrack

This type is capable of recording (and playing back) many independent audio tracks. Tape based systems, whether analog or digital, are traditionally available as four-track (e.g. 8-track, 16-track, or 24-track multiples). Digital tape multitracks are typically modular eight-track units—if more tracks are required, more individual units are bought and linked together. With analog tape, the width of each physical audio track will have an affect on the overall quality of the recorded signal, with wider being better. Multitracks are used in the capture and production of audio when there are many sound sources requiring independent editing and control, and they are not really used in the generation of a final "product" as two-tracks are. Modern *nonlinear* multitrack devices are now capable of almost limitless numbers of audio tracks.

Linear

Tape (analog or digital) is linear in that information is laid sequentially onto the medium with increasing time (as is CD-R). The only way that this information can be rearranged is by physically cutting and splicing sections of tape (although some digital tape systems allow rudimentary offline editing facilities). Tape based systems need to have transport mechanisms to fast forward or rewind to specific points, hence taking some time to move around the medium. CD/CD-R does similarly but, due to the nature of the medium, has much quicker seek and access times.

Nonlinear

Minidisk and hard disk recording systems store and access information from all over the surface of the medium, with the implication that seek times are virtually instantaneous, and editing becomes much easier to handle.

Digital Audio Workstation

This is a modern computer based recorder/editor that is effectively a software program running on a computing device that supports at least two-track audio input and output, with the system hard disk being used as the actual recording medium. The notion of "tracks" therefore becomes somewhat redundant as they are merely a particular type of data file to be loaded, edited, and saved by the computer hardware/software, although now containing audio information rather than, for instance, text. Hence, these systems are digital, nonlinear, multitrack devices (even if they only physically support two audio inputs and outputs, many internal virtual tracks will be available for simultaneous playback of multiple instruments or takes). Audio editing becomes as easy as editing a text document in a word processor, and the files used are capable of being stored in many different formats, with many possible combinations of sample rate and bit resolution, although 16/24 bit, 44.1/48 kHz WAV, and AIFF are some of those most commonly encountered. Stereo and mono files are supported readily, and some file formats also support multiple audio channels, as used for instance in some surround-sound formats. When working with audio files, sample rate considerations are as before and 24-bit resolution should be used wherever possible (although not readily supported by most basic computer audio inputs/outputs, the software should be able to deal with this format readily). Note also that WAV and AIFF files use no data compression so all information is stored exactly as it is recorded.

MP3 and other similar files use perceptually based *data compression* schemes to reduce the physical size of the audio data file, while delivering audio playback that "sounds the same" as the original uncompressed version. Such compressed files should be avoided when recording and editing at all costs to maintain signal integrity and quality, and some systems might use such a recording mode as an optional or default setting. However MP3 (and similar) are useful for distribution of audio material across the Internet as they are quick to upload and download, and good quality can be maintained with appropriate encoder settings; however, the uncompressed source files should always be maintained for future reference.

VOCAL SOUND REINFORCEMENT

Introduction

So far, this chapter has discussed the background theory behind microphone selection for vocal work and how this signal might be further manipulated using standard audio hardware (or software) prior to, or as part of, the recording and mixing/production process. The microphones and equipment discussed so far are common to many application areas, both research and commercially focused, with their most obvious use being in vocal recording. However, there is one important area not covered so far that has very different and specific requirements, and that is vocal amplification, more generally called *sound reinforcement*. The purpose of such a system is to amplify a signal that may otherwise be too quiet or too far away to be heard effectively by the intended audience, so that it is perceived as being louder or closer. A sound reinforcement system will therefore consist of everything discussed so far—microphones to capture acoustic signals, mixing desks and effects to manipulate these signals further, perhaps with an additional multitrack recording medium—but now also with the addition of amplifiers and loudspeakers. Clearly these devices will also be used at the signal capture/recording stage, at the most basic level via headphones, but the purpose of sound reinforcement in this context is quite different. Here the signals must be projected, usually at significant levels, over some distance so that both performers and audience can hear the results to their individual satisfaction. Needless to say there are major problems that prevent this from being a trivial process. Therefore, with microphones connected to the inputs of a mixer, which will also have connections to additional sound processing options, it is necessary to connect to the mixer outputs an amplification and loudspeaker system. This combination of microphone/mixer/amp/speaker gives the basic definition of a sound reinforcement system, also very commonly known as a PA, or *public address system*. They are found in many different scenarios and application areas, from announcement systems in shops, railway stations, and public spaces, in lecture halls, outside radio broadcast and theaters, through to the large, highly complex systems used at major indoor and outdoor concert venues. In fact, anywhere a person's voice needs to be heard where it could not possibly be otherwise without the intervention of some means of artificial help. What follows is a brief introduction to the equipment and principles of

sound reinforcement through the consideration of different sized systems, together with some general guidelines for their operation.

Small Venues

A basic PA system is shown in Figure 4–21, where performers and loudspeakers are mounted on a stage, facing an audience. The main mixing desk (often called the *front-of-house* [FOH] mixing desk) is placed usually in the middle of the auditorium at the ideal listening position where a sound engineer will operate it and be able to judge the quality of the overall sound that the audience will be hearing. In reality it is often the case in smaller venues that the desk is placed wherever there is space for it, as not all situations are ideal. Some PA systems, for instance for solo performers, are designed to be operated without a separate sound engineer and may actually be located on the stage. Although a convenient necessity, it does imply that making changes mid-performance or judging what the audience will be hearing is difficult.

Most of this system should be familiar from what has been discussed in this chapter so far:

■ Microphones are used to capture a performance, either vocal or instrumental.
■ The microphones are connected to a mixing desk for further manipulation and mixing.
■ The mixing desk will make use of additional optional insert and send/return effects.
■ A main mix is constructed via the main mix L/R outputs.

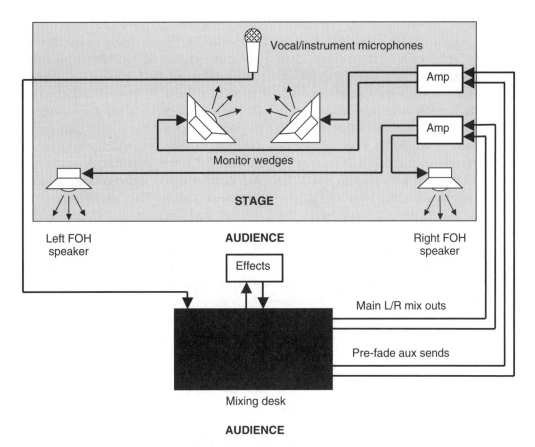

Figure 4–21. *A basic PA system suitable for small to medium sized venues.*

- Pre-fade aux sends are used to construct foldback mixes for the performers.

The main change to this basic system is the addition of amplification (amps) and loudspeakers, how they are used, and their arrangement on the stage.

The FOH PA system is used to project the amplified sound of the performers across the audience. Loudspeakers are arranged to the left and right of the stage area corresponding to stereo left and right, although it is worth noting that the very simplest PA systems may only produce a single mono output, in which case it is not possible to pan a sound on the mixing desk as both loudspeakers will produce the same common acoustic signal. The amplifiers work similarly to the gain control at the input to the channel of the mixing desk, except on a much larger scale. The low level signal produced by the mixing desk outputs has to be boosted many times so that it is suitable for driving the large FOH loudspeakers and producing enough acoustic sound energy to enable the signal to be heard at a sufficient volume level across the venue. PA systems are therefore rated in watts (W) or kilowatts (kW), determining the maximum continuous power handling limitation of the system. Small venues, conferences, or vocal only systems may need somewhere in the region of 100 to 300 W, whereas if a vocal signal needs to compete with loud or amplified instruments such as drums or electric guitar, a 300 to 500 W system would be more appropriate. For larger venues, club DJs, or larger bands a 1000 W (1 kW) system would be a good starting point. Outdoor PA systems for large concerts may be in the region of 10 kW. As a rule, the higher the power rating of the PA system, the more headroom will be available when mixing—that is, the easier it will be to make the audio signal heard across the venue without running into the danger of clipping distortion or "blowing" a speaker by driving it too hard.

Note that on the simplest PA systems, the amps may well be combined with the loudspeaker enclosures themselves, being quick to set up, easy to transport, and generally convenient to use. In other systems, the amplifiers may be combined with the mixing desk. Both options allow for some system scalability, with the former allowing any mixing desk to be used with the powered speakers, and the latter allowing for the speakers themselves to be upgraded or replaced cheaply and easily.

The *monitor* system is the means by which the performers are allowed to hear themselves as they play. This is particularly important for vocalists; whereas some instruments such as a drum kit or electric guitar produce sufficient level for the musicians to hear themselves over the general sound produced by the FOH PA system, the voice source will only be amplified by the FOH system itself, which is designed to point forwards and away from the performer,

projecting the audio signal out across the audience. Hence, traditional monitor systems consist of loudspeakers built into wedge shaped enclosures (hence the term *monitor wedges*) such that when placed on the floor they are designed to point backwards and upwards at the vocalist. In the system demonstrated in Figure 4–21 the monitor wedges are driven by a signal sourced from the pre-fade aux sends. This means that the content and level of this signal can be controlled completely separately from the signal being sent to the FOH system and are not affected by any settings or changes made to the main channel faders that determine the main FOH L/R mix. The vocal performer may then wish for a particular balance of signals for her own personal monitor mix—perhaps just a little electric guitar together with a significant amount of her own vocal signal—and using this method, such independent level and content control is possible. For small venues or small PA systems, it is often the case that only the vocal performance will be run through the system; the other instruments may be capable of producing an appropriate signal level without any additional sound reinforcement. The only problem with such a simple setup is that it would be impossible to give the vocalist (or other performer) a monitor mix consisting of anything other than vocals. Hence, for complete control over the monitor mix, all instruments should be run via the desk, even if they are not used directly in the main FOH mix. Finally, as with the FOH system, the most basic monitoring systems usually combine the amplification and loudspeaker stages as part of the monitor wedge for simplicity and convenience.

Medium Sized Venues

A larger or more complex sound reinforcement system may be required for
one or more of the following reasons:

■ There may be a need to project sound
over a larger venue or audience.
■ The use of more on-stage performers
may necessitate greater flexibility
and control over monitor mixing.
■ To facilitate better monitoring and
FOH mixing, all performers have to
be run through the mixing desk.

■ It will produce general improvements in the overall FOH sound
quality.

Figure 4–22 demonstrates such a
system and, by comparison with Figure
4–21, it should be clear that there is significant commonality between the two.
There are two main differences, one of
which is that there are now more monitor wedges used, each with independent
control via a pre-fade auxiliary send. This,
together with the larger number of performers—and therefore microphones—

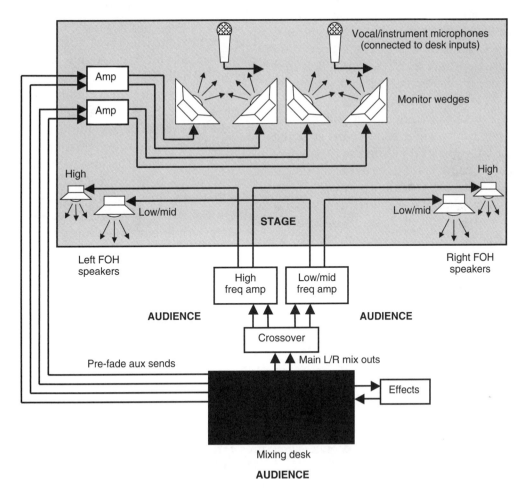

Figure 4–22. *A typical PA system suitable for medium sized venues.*

possibly being accommodated, would imply that the number of cables running between the mixing desk and the stage will start to become non-trivial. Hence a *multicore* and *breakout box* (sometimes also called a *snake*) arrangement is typically used. A multicore is basically a long and thick cable that carries within it many individual signal cables. At either end of the multicore cable is a breakout box consisting of individual audio connectors wired into these individual cable strands. Due to the long distances multicores are typically used over, and the increased possibility of signal problems due to induced noise or interference as the individual cables are very tightly packed together, multicores are designed to carry balanced signals and hence male/female XLR connectors are used at the breakout boxes.

The second difference is in the use of a *crossover*. Larger PA systems split the audio signal into different frequency bands using a series of electrical filters, and different types of loudspeaker are used to handle each frequency band according to what design is best suited to the task. In Figure 4–22, the crossover splits the audio signal into two, consisting of a high frequency and combined low/mid range frequency band. Such an example would be found in most basic PA speaker cabinets where (for instance) a 15-inch bass/mid speaker is combined with a much smaller (1- to 3-inch) speaker, often called a *tweeter*. A *passive crossover* splits the signal after it has been amplified, usually within the speaker housing, and is a technique commonly found in domestic hi-fi systems. They are usually economical and reliable, and are best suited for low output systems. An *active crossover* splits the signal before it reaches the amplifiers, and are gener-

ally more suitable for higher output and higher quality systems, although as more channels of amplification are required, are more expensive and complicated to use. The example shown in Figure 4–22 has the crossover before the amplifiers and is therefore an example of an active crossover.

Large Venues/More Complex Sound Reinforcement Systems

The next level of complexity, suitable for the largest venues, large stages, and many performers/instrumentalists, is to separate the FOH mixing from the on-stage monitor mixing. This gives much more control of the on-stage sound balance and will usually allow each performer to have her own individual monitor mix. Most standard FOH mixing desks will also start to run out of pre-fade auxiliary sends, and so a dedicated monitor mixing desk is required. This arrangement is demonstrated in Figure 4–23, although note that only four monitor wedges are shown for clarity. The microphone signals are sent to both FOH and monitor desks via a splitter, and in this case via multicore cables. Finally, a three-way active crossover is employed, consisting now of a tweeter for high frequencies, a mid-range speaker, and a large *subwoofer* for the very lowest bass frequencies, typically below 120 Hz.

Operational Guidelines

With the fundamental aspects of a sound reinforcement system defined, and hopefully in place in a venue, it is important to consider some basic operating principles. What follows are therefore guidelines that can be applied in most PA appli-

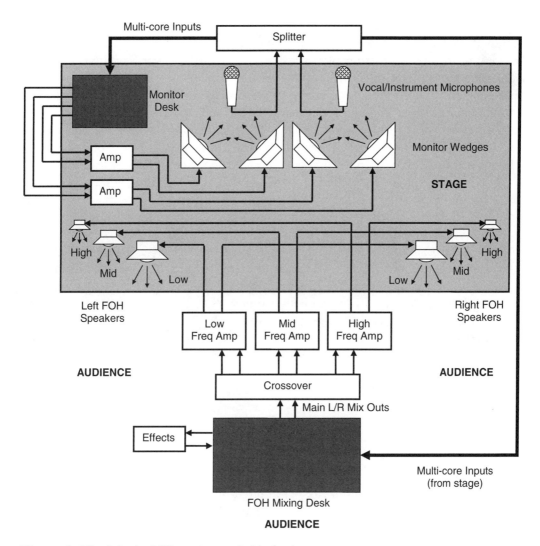

Figure 4–23. *A typical PA system suitable for large venues.*

cations and will help the beginner to achieve a good overall balance of sound while minimizing potential problems. However, no matter how helpful they may be, these guidelines should not be considered as a replacement for practice, experience, and careful listening skills.

General Setup and Speaker Positioning

It is important to turn up for such an event as early as possible. This allows plenty of time for considering the venue and where equipment should be located, for running cables from desk to stage, and troubleshooting possible problems. If the PA is already installed, it will give time to get familiar with the system. In both cases it should allow time for a sound check to let both performers and engineers become familiar with this particular venue and setup.

Speakers should be mounted to the left and right of the stage such that they project out over the audience, so use stands if available or stack the speakers to an appropriate level using platforms or staging blocks. This of course implies that for safety, both floor and stands should be rigid and secure. The most important aspect is to have them as far forward in front of the main microphones as is possible, thereby preventing FOH sound from being picked up by the stage microphones, particularly the vocal microphones, leading to problems with feedback (see below). Angle the speakers if possible or appropriate so that they don't directly point at large surfaces in the room, such as the side or rear walls, which would cause problematic reflections and lead to possible sound quality or feedback problems. It is also helpful in some venues to point speakers away from where people might be working—for instance a bar area—and to ensure that fire exits or entrances are not blocked. Similarly, cable runs should be placed away from points of ingress or egress to avoid potential trip hazards.

The main mixing desk and associated equipment should ideally be placed at the midpoint between left and right speakers and in the center of the audience. In this way the sound engineer is ideally placed to hear the stereo balance, to get a good idea as to what most of the audience will be hearing, and to have good eye contact with the on-stage performers. Often in smaller venues this can be difficult to achieve and so a compromise has to be reached. Eye contact to facilitate communication might actually be the most important option to consider here; in such venues it is relatively easy to take a quick walk around the audience area during sound check and sometimes during the performance as well to listen to what will be heard and make adjustments to suit back at the desk.

Monitor speakers can be very problematic in terms of feedback, as they will be projecting sound back towards the performers and hence the microphones. They should again be positioned carefully. Wedge monitors will often be positioned incorrectly, especially if on-stage space is at a premium as it usually is in smaller venues; they should point at the ears of the performers relative to where they are standing, not at their knees! Acoustic reflections are also problematic if there are hard, flat surfaces around the on-stage area—sound projected from the monitors will reflect off these surfaces and quite possibly arrive back at the front of the microphone. Again, careful positioning can help to minimize such potential problems. Drapes, soft materials, or even a banner with the band/artist name on it can help to provide additional acoustic absorption across a large, flat wall behind the performers and help to cut down on reflected sound energy. It is also important to know what microphone types are being used, particularly by a vocalist, who will require good monitoring, usually from wedges. A cardioid pattern microphone has the null point at the rear. Therefore, to avoid sound pickup from the monitors they should be placed directly in front of the microphone. Hypercardioids and supercardioids have two null points off to either side. In such a situation monitor speakers should be moved offset from center to coincide with these null points.

Unfortunately, in a situation where there are many performers grouped closely together, particularly if some of them are using acoustically loud or amplified instruments such as drums or electric guitar, *spill* can be a problem, particularly with vocal microphones. This is where signals other than the desired source are picked up by a specific microphone. Getting the vocalist to use the microphone close in can help, but again positioning is often the key so that vocalists are not placed directly in front of louder instruments. Reflections from the rear wall of the stage area can also cause problems relating to spill, and positioning additional strategically placed absorption across such surfaces can again help to alleviate this.

Feedback Elimination

Probably the biggest problem that will be faced is that of acoustic feedback; this occurs when the signal from a loudspeaker is picked up by a microphone that then in turn sends the signal back through the desk/PA system to the same amp/loudspeaker combination, where it will be amplified further, projected, and picked up by the same microphone again. A *feedback loop* is created, and the gain of the signal in the loop rapidly increases, resulting in the typical high-pitched ringing or squealing sound that is hated by both audience and artist alike. The pitch or frequency of this sound is determined by factors such as the resonant frequencies of the microphone, amplifier, and loudspeaker, the acoustics of the room, the directional properties of the loudspeaker and microphone, and the distance between them. The more gain that is applied to a signal, the more likely it is that feedback will occur.

A vocalist with poor voice projection, and/or who is at some distance from the microphone, will need a significant amount of gain to be applied at the mixer input to bring the signal up to a useful level. The additional gain applied

will increase the likelihood of feedback on this channel. Hence, good microphone technique and vocal technique are important for minimizing feedback. The vocalist should also never put hands around the microphone grill. Remember that the directional characteristic of a microphone is determined by allowing the acoustic signal to arrive at the diaphragm from both in front and behind the microphone. If the grill is cupped in the singer's hands, the rear access vents will be blocked, effectively making the microphone omnidirectional. Similarly, it is almost second nature, if a vocalist hears feedback, to put a hand over the front of the microphone with the aim of trying to stop it; of course, sound will still enter from the rearwards path, and all that is done with this action is to make the microphone more omnidirectional and therefore even more prone to feedback problems! Microphone technique in this context also includes the use of handheld microphones and the performer being aware how her on-stage movements might influence possible feedback problems related to the location of the PA FOH and monitoring loudspeakers.

Careful positioning of loudspeakers (FOH and monitor) and microphones is the most important point to consider when trying to eliminate possible causes of feedback, as has already been discussed above. This should be done with due consideration of the polar pickup pattern of the microphones being used. Potential sources of strong acoustic reflections also need to be considered and eliminated wherever possible, and it can also help to make sure that monitors and microphone stands are not too close together; the vibrations of a speaker cabinet can be transmitted through the floor and stand to the microphone itself, providing a mechanical coupling of source and receiver that can also then lead to acoustic feedback. Carpet or rubber matting under the monitors can help if this does seem to be a problem.

Feedback problems caused due to the FOH speaker system can be fairly easily dealt with using the above checks. However, feedback caused by the monitor speakers can be much more problematic, particularly if the venue or stage is small and there is little room for adequate spacing or positioning of microphones or monitor wedges. The key here is to connect a graphic EQ (see section on Conditioning the Signal Further—Inserts and EQ) between the mixing desk monitor feed and the monitor or monitor amp. Graphic EQs have many narrow bands of frequency cut/boost and these can be used to "ring out" specific regions of the spectrum that are prone to feedback. Practice and experience allow a sound engineer to do this quickly, but with enough time before the sound check and some patience it is easy for those with only basic expertise to accomplish:

- Place the main vocal microphone in a stand in its typical on-stage position.
- With the monitor system on and the vocal microphone channel being routed to the nearest monitor speakers, turn up the gain for this channel until on the verge of feedback. This should be easy to hear— there will be the very quietest hint of the typical feedback ring, and even the slightest increase in channel gain will result in it becoming very loud indeed.
- With the microphone/monitors on the verge of feeding back like this, turn to the graphic EQ. Starting at the lowest frequency band, very slightly *increase* the gain on the slider— 3–6 dB should be more than enough —and then return it to 0 dB. Most frequency bands will have no affect when doing this (although note that any frequency band will feedback if the gain slider is turned up too much—care and subtlety are the key!), but the band closest to the most problematic resonant frequency in the system will result in almost immediate dramatic feedback. This is the offending frequency, and therefore this slider should be turned *down* on the graphic EQ by about 6 dB.
- With the first problem frequency identified and now "notched out," the channel gain can be turned up a little more until the system is again on the verge of feeding back. The same process of identification and elimination can then be applied.

It is worth doing this for the first few problematic frequencies. Typically, they will be in the low end of the spectrum and should not affect the general sound quality of what is coming through the monitors too much. However, if this is done right through the spectrum, and given that even the best graphic EQ will still have sliders with a third-octave bandwidth, the overall timbre will be changed considerably. Every time a graphic EQ slider is turned down, part of the original source signal is removed, and clearly this is not ideal. However, there is more room for such timbre change with the monitoring system, as it is only there as a reference for the performers, than there is should the FOH system need to be rung out in a similar manner due to really bad feedback problems with the main loudspeakers. As a final word of warning when using graphic EQs, it is very easy to knock a frequency band cut/boost slider by accident without noticing, or to have them ever so slightly off from their 0 dB point. Even a few dB of unwanted gain could cause feedback, so ensure that all such unwanted bands are absolutely at 0 dB. This is generally easy to check, as the slider will be notched at this point so that it moves into place with a click that can be felt. Also make sure that the careful ringing out of the monitor (or FOH) system hasn't resulted in nearly all of the frequency bands being attenuated slightly—as well as being undesirable in terms of timbre, the overall effect will be the same as having just turned the gain controls for the speaker channel down by the same amount. Graphic EQs shouldn't be used as glorified volume controls! Finally, some monitor wedges also come with basic low/mid/high EQ controls for performers to adjust the sound to suit their preference. The hard work done in ringing out a system can be undone if the performer decides to change these controls mid–performance; hence, communication with the performers during sound check is important so that all parties are aware of the system being used and are happy with the sound being achieved. Also, check if these controls are set incorrectly or have been accidentally knocked, as this could be the source of hard-to-remove feedback.

Additional signal processing can also help with particularly problematic feedback. It can be tempting to apply compression to the main vocal to make it "sit above" the overall mix. Although desirable from a music production standpoint, this is actually dangerous to do in terms of feedback. It may give a profes-

sional studio sound, and allow the overall level of the vocal to rise a few extra dB, but the dynamics of the performance will be lost, and most importantly in this context, the level of the quieter aspects of the signal will be boosted. This potentially includes those frequencies that are prone to feedback that otherwise wouldn't be; therefore, compression should be used with some care on individual instruments, although generally a little stereo compression over the main left/right FOH mix can help with the overall sound and prevent tweeters from being blown by accidental signal peaks or unexpected feedback. Noise gates can be used and will help to reduce spill and possible feedback problems when the microphone is "open"—that is, turned up at the desk and turned on—but not being used by the vocalist or performer at that point in a piece. However in this case, care must be taken with the gate settings to ensure that aspects of the performance are not lost, such as the start or end of words or quieter moments. Finally, specific feedback suppression units can be connected between desk and amp/loudspeaker. These consist of banks of narrowband notch filters that automatically ring out the PA system to a ready state, and can then also react to problematic frequencies that might feedback during the performance. If feedback is detected, a filter will lock on to the problematic frequency and attenuate it automatically. Such a device doesn't stop feedback completely as it has to occur and be detected before it can be removed, but it does offer a layer of insurance during the performance and is usually quicker than a human finger on the fader. Feedback suppressors also do obviously affect the timbre of the sound, and this can be undesirable, again especially if they are used on the FOH system, but this is generally more acceptable to engineers, audience, and performers than listening to the feedback itself.

Sound Check and Level Management

With efforts having been made as much as possible to eliminate possible sources of feedback, the full system should be ready for sound checking. It is often useful at this point to run a CD player (or something similar) through a couple of spare channels of the desk so that signal input/output can be checked and a general level set. It also helps to have a microphone connected to the main mixing desk on a spare channel at the FOH position; this allows the engineer to communicate with the performers via the monitor speakers. All instruments should be checked first, whether miked up or directly connected to the desk, and then vocal microphones should be checked. With most performances, it is the vocal, whether sung or spoken, that is the most important aspect, carrying the message for the audience (whether artistic or factual), being their focal point and demanding their attention. Hence, once it has been established that all of the connected acoustic/electric sources are working correctly, the overall level should be set with reference to the main vocal source. A useful way to establish this is as follows:

- Turn down all the vocal microphone channel gain controls.
- Set the master output L/R mix fader to about two thirds its maximum value.
- Set the microphone channel faders at maximum so that they are boosting

the signal above the usual unity gain, 0 dB, setting.
- Slowly turn up the vocal channel gain control until it is just at the point of feedback (as when ringing out the system) and then back it off slightly so that any ringing can no longer be heard.
- Bring the vocal microphone channel faders back to 0 dB and balance all the other instruments to this level.

This procedure sets a good working level for the vocals, with about 10 dB of safe headroom where they can be boosted further without danger of feeding back. There is also similar room for altering the overall mix level, either cutting or boosting according to the demands of the venue or the performance. A similar procedure can be used to set the levels of the monitor speakers.

The sound check performs many functions: it allows the performers to warm up and ensure they are happy with their own setup and the PA system in general, it allows the engineer to do a full system check, levels can be set and tested, an overall balance can be achieved, etc. It is important at this stage to ensure the performers are happy with what is being heard on-stage, and that working monitor mixes are established, depending on how many speakers and speaker feeds there are and what each performer wishes to hear. The desk should also be annotated using marking tape and pen to label channels, groups, and auxiliaries, and it can be helpful to use a wax pencil or nonpermanent marker to set reference level marks for the channel faders. Visual communication between performers and engineer is critical so that changes can be made on the fly during a performance. Obviously, under these circumstances the engineer should not use the microphone routed to the monitors as it may give the performers a surprise midsong, and similarly it is not very professional for vocal performers to request changes via the main FOH system so that the entire audience can hear.

Finally, despite every check, balance, and test as part of the sound check, there is every possibility that the whole system will need to be adjusted with an audience in the venue. They will helpfully act to absorb some of the acoustic energy projected into the space, including possibly problematic reflections or feedback paths, and as a result, the overall level may need to be pushed slightly higher. Also, the immediate interaction between performer and audience will generally push the musicians/performers to a different level of performance from that in a simple rehearsal or sound check, often with a rise in acoustic output and individual signal levels. Hence, be ready to bring these levels down slightly if there is a danger of feedback or overloading distortion.

SUMMARY

This chapter has introduced the technology required to capture, condition, process, mix, and amplify an acoustic signal, focusing mainly on the vocal source, either spoken or sung. The performer and reader should now have a working understanding as to the basic operating principles of a microphone, and what might influence microphone selection for a particular vocal recording or sound reinforcement task. The next step in this chain is the connection of the selected microphone to a mixing desk and routing and preparing the signal ready for recording, mixing, or amplification. This includes the basics of EQ and effects processing, including compression, gating, and reverberation. The concept of the recording medium has been introduced, and finally this chapter has considered the fundamentals of sound reinforcement and PA systems, including a guide to the basic operating principles. With this knowledge in place, the next chapter will ex-plore how it might be applied in a variety of common vocal recording scenarios.

FURTHER READING

Bartlett, B., & Bartlett, J. (2005). *Practical recording techniques: The step-by-step approach to professional audio recording* (4th ed.). Oxford, UK: Focal Press.

Bohn, D. A. (1986, September). Constant-Q graphic equalizers. *Journal of the Audio Engineering Society, 34*, 611–626.

Eargle, J. (2004). *The microphone book: From mono to stereo to surround—A guide to microphone design and application* (2nd ed.). Oxford, UK: Focal Press.

Howard, D. M., & Angus, J. A. S. (2006). *Acoustics and psychoacoustics* (3rd ed.). Oxford, UK: Focal Press.

Rumsey, F., & McCormick, T. (2005). *Sound and recording—An introduction* (5th ed.). Oxford, UK: Focal Press.

Sundberg, J. (1992). *The science of musical sounds.* : Elsevier.

Talbot-Smith, M. (2004). *Sound engineering explained* (2nd ed.). Oxford, UK: Focal Press.

Talbot-Smith, M. (2004). *Sound engineer's pocket book* (2nd ed.). Oxford, UK: Focal Press.

CHAPTER 5

Practical Voice Recording and Reinforcement

With the previous chapter having established the concepts, terms, and technology related to voice recording and sound reinforcement, this knowledge is now applied to a number of common vocal recording/reinforcement scenarios. It is worth noting that although the previous chapter considered a typical full studio/live setup, it is also possible to get good quality vocal recordings from a simple microphone and portable digital recorder combination. However, such devices do work on the same principles as those discussed at length in Chapter 4, and hence terms such as sample rate, bit resolution, level, dynamic range, clipping, etc., remain entirely relevant. It is also worth checking with portable recorders that they support external microphones and are capable of supplying phantom power to allow the use of condenser mikes. There may also be other limitations (in terms of features or sound quality), so thorough testing, checking, and listening to test recordings

is advised prior to making a critical recording. Hence, setting up a simple microphone/recorder arrangement and capturing a vocal in a "quick and dirty" fashion is easy to do and good results can be achieved. This chapter aims to improve on this basic premise by offering suitable guidelines for making high quality, professional recordings in a number of different scenarios with little additional preparation or effort. These scenarios will include common studio, live, commercial, or research examples and introduce more advanced techniques such as creating high quality, natural stereo recordings. All of these examples will be approached by considering three fundamental elements.

Source

Consider first, and most importantly, the nature of the vocal source. Is it a solo voice or does it consist of multiple sources? This will, for instance, dictate the number of microphones required, and their type. Is the source spoken or sung? Is the lead voice male or female or a balanced mix of both? What backing, in terms of either music or general background sound/noise, will accompany the voice? Is it possible or desirable to position microphones close to the source, or must they be out of sight? Listen also to the sound quality of the voice—is it for instance particularly sibilant? Are there any other problems or features that you should make a note of?

Location

Next consider the environment in which the recording is going to take place. Is it possible to exert some control over this—can the time and location of the recording session be altered to suit? Is the space large or small, reverberant or very dry sounding? If there are some imposed limitations, then what can be learned or anticipated about the characteristics of the recording space that might be optimized or compensated for? These characteristics might extend to the surroundings of the space—is it outside or inside? What are the chances of extraneous noise interfering with the actual recording process? Such noise may be present all the time, such as air conditioning (Could it be turned off?) or traffic noise (recording at night might be quieter) or only on certain occasions, such as church bells chiming the hour—again, could they be turned off?

Listener

Rather than the individual(s) listening to the recording, this refers to what the recording is to be used for. A fully produced pop record will have different requirements from a classical choral recording. Live vocal sound reinforcement will have its own set of limitations or requirements, and a loud pop concert will differ again from simple spoken public address. Recording voice for research or analysis purposes will also have very different and unique requirements compared to commercial or performance based recording applications. Hence, it is fundamentally important to consider the application to which the final vocal recording will be put. Where will it finally end up, how will it be auditioned, who will be doing the auditioning, and why?

In all of the above stages it is important to consider these issues before the session commences; otherwise, less-than-ideal equipment for the recording might have to be used, or the outcome might require extensive editing to make it useful for the intended listener—if it can be fixed at all. A phrase often used in recording circles is to "fix it in the mix." This means that if there is a problem with the actual recording (in terms of performance, sound, noise, or any of the other problems that might occur) it is easy to rectify the problem through post-recording mixing, editing, and judicious use of audio processing. Although this might work on some occasions, it is no guarantee and no replacement for getting the sound right at source with good microphone selection and technique. It is also often a false economy as editing and processing after the event will usually take longer than just getting the recording right at source.

This chapter is divided into two sections, dividing possible sources into two groups, consisting of single vocal sources and multiple vocal sources, and thereby considering relevant case studies separately under these headings. Each scenario will then be introduced and dealt with according to the three points introduced above and in light of what has been covered in Chapter 4. The section on multiple sources will also include an introduction to stereo recording techniques.

SINGLE VOCAL SOURCES

Introduction

This chapter section deals with recording or reinforcing the solo voice, which may be speech or singing. Generally, the desire with this range of applications is to capture the vocal source as cleanly and directly as possible, in such a way that all other surrounding sources, including noise, and reverberation are sufficiently attenuated to the point that they are no longer of any concern. All that matters is the dry, direct sound emanating from the vocal source. When such a recording is auditioned directly it will sound very close and unnatural, as we are generally used to hearing sounds in the context of the acoustic space in which they are placed. However, capturing just the dry sound in this way gives clean raw material for the researcher to analyze and maximum flexibility to the producer/composer/engineer during the post-recording process. Editing becomes easier, various creative and corrective effects processes can be applied, and different types of artificial reverberation and spatial processing can be applied and experimented with.

Recording for Research

Whereas for most recording or sound reinforcement applications it is sufficient to place a microphone in front of a vocalist and get a "good sound," for research applications additional rigor is required in terms of the final listener to establish the validity of any results produced and to remove possible sources of experimental error. To capture the vocal source, a "transparent sounding" microphone is required to ensure that the effect of the microphone's own frequency response on the spectral content of the voice is minimized as much as possible. Therefore, wherever possible, an omnidirectional condenser microphone should be used due to its high sensitivity and extended flat frequency response.

The location for the recording may be a problem, although every opportunity should be taken to ensure that such critical work is carried out in an anechoic chamber (see section, Anechoic Recording) or at least a controlled studio environment (see section, Studio Vocal Recording). If there are noise problems, or the recording room is very reverberant, action will be needed to ensure that these signal components do not interfere too much with the actual voice source once recorded. In a more commercial recording application, the obvious answer would be to select a directional microphone such as a cardioid. However, the problem here is the very non-flat frequency response of such microphones, which is far from ideal when a true representation of the voice is required. The best option would be to use a small head-mounted microphone. These are often omnidirectional (although it is important to check) and hence will have a good flat frequency response and give remarkably acceptable results. A directional microphone should be used only as a last resort, and at an appropriate distance to minimize any possible proximity effect.

Assuming that an omnidirectional microphone is being used, the next important consideration is to calibrate the device in terms of sound pressure level (SPL). Specific high quality measurement microphones will often come with an SPL calibrator for this purpose, and they are designed to produce a specific SPL, for instance 94 dB at 1 kHz (although some are capable of higher SPL values but at lower frequencies), when attached to the front of the microphone. However, these are usually only designed to be used with the microphone they come with, as they have to fit closely around the front of the capsule, and should never be used on a directional microphone. There are other ways to calibrate the microphone, however. One method is to play a 1 kHz test-tone at 94 db SPL from a loudspeaker, using an SPL meter to check for the correct acoustic signal level. The minimum source to microphone distance is 30 cm, and these distances should always be measured accurately and noted down, as an SPL calibration is useless without it. A headset microphone can be calibrated similarly by adjusting its level, once in position, to match that of an SPL meter at a distance from the source, e.g., at 30 cm. A long sustained vowel sound can be used as the test source in this case, rather than a pre-prepared test-tone signal. This automatically accounts for the short source-microphone distance and will give results as if the recordings were made at 30 cm distance. Similarly, for such research applications it is always important to note general distances and placements of sources, microphones, etc., so that experiments can be repeated if required and reported accurately.

Finally, in terms of location, it is always important to place the microphone within the *critical distance* or *reverberation radius* of the room, to ensure that the direct sound dominates over the reflected reverberation. If it is required to capture low level acoustic signals, a much shorter distance (or alternatively a headset microphone) might be appropriate. Source and microphone should also be placed away from possible reflecting surfaces such as walls, windows, or even such items as music stands, as the reflected sound will be picked up by the microphone, coloring the timbre of the original source recording.

Studio Vocal Recording

This is a common scenario that offers the potential for high quality, controlled results, where the singer is usually isolated from the engineer and studio control room. Typically, the goal here is to capture the source—male/female, singing, or spoken—in isolation from all other aspects, including other performers, noise, reverberation etc. Generally the source in this context will be the focal point for the final listener—it may be the lead vocal of a song, a voiceover for a film soundtrack, or a museum audio guide. It is also quite possible that the studio location is used to record the voice for research purposes due to the controlled acoustic that is usually offered. However, for nonresearch purposes, calibration is not so important as is the need to capture the natural performance offered by the vocalist as transparently and easily as possible. It is therefore important to remember that the performer might not be used to such a recording environment where he is essentially removed from all other direct contact and then observed closely through a glass window from the studio control room. Hence, to be able to capture the best performance it is important to put the vocalist at ease and accommodate his wishes as much as possible. Perhaps the most important aspect here is communication, which is facilitated via the actual vocal microphone used and the vocalist's headphones, through which a foldback mix is delivered (see Chapter 4, section Interfacing with External Devices—The Auxiliary Section). Communication from control room to performer is facilitated through the mixing desk talkback facility, where pressing the talkback button activates a small microphone on the mixing desk, picking up any speech and transmitting it through to the foldback headphones. To keep performers at ease, it is good practice to keep up good communication via this facility, even if they are not involved directly with control room activities— for instance, when signals are being rerouted or patched via different cables. It is also very easy to talk away to the performer in the other room without realizing the talkback button is not pressed, particularly if there is more than one person present in the control room.

A good foldback mix is also important, and again the wishes of the performer should be accommodated as he might not want to hear the same balance of instruments as the control room engineer. It is also commonly accepted that adding a small amount of reverb to the vocal, and routing this through to the foldback mix, will help a singer to stay more in tune. If a singer does like this option it is important to double check that the reverberated source signal is not the one that is recorded; only the direct, dry signal should be committed to permanent record at this stage, as reverbs can be added, edited, and adjusted to suit when mixing/editing but cannot be changed if captured at source.

Most studio recording spaces offer a controlled acoustic environment, isolated from all external noise sources, with quiet air conditioning systems. It might be possible to alter the reverberation present in the room and hence captured on the recording via movable panels, drapes, or location within the room itself (some spaces have "live ends" and "dead ends," giving some variability in the amount of potential reverberation offered), but when capturing a single vocal source in this manner, a dry, nonreverberated sound is required so that this can be added later at the editing/mixing stage. In non-ideal spaces, or on occasions where there may be other performers present, reverberation, reflections, or spill should be minimized through careful source placement or use of drapes, acoustic panels, or portable isolation booths/panels and of course good microphone technique. Even in the best spaces, as with research focused recording, it is important to beware of possibly troublesome reflections from hard, flat surfaces, as this delayed version of the direct signal adds to the original to cause timbral coloration in a process called *phase cancellation*. Control room windows, walls, doors, and music stands are all possible causes of such reflections, and so source and microphone should be positioned accordingly.

Microphone Choice and Positioning

A flat condenser microphone with a large diaphragm is the generally best option —or, alternatively, the most expensive of the microphones that are available. This will give an extended frequency bandwidth and offer considerable sensitivity and minimal additional extraneous noise. However, if time permits, it is always a good idea to try out a range of microphones to arrive at one to suit the individual performer. By making some test recordings, the performer can also help in the decision-making process by listening to how the final result will sound, with the additional consequence of this being the development of trust between engineer and vocalist before the session starts. If the final listener is expecting a male voice to appear as part of a rock song, a dynamic cardioid microphone might deliver the sound required for this particular session. If the vocalist is particularly sibilant, a dynamic microphone might also be favored, although there are other ways to get around this problem as discussed below.

The best polar pickup pattern depends upon the acoustics of the room and the position and level of any other sound sources within it. A cardioid is usually the default choice and will give an intimate feel. An omnidirectional pattern will give a more open, natural, and transparent sound, and again allowing some time for experimentation will pay dividends. The microphone itself should also be checked for specific settings. Attenuation or padding should not be required, and check if there is a low-cut filter on the microphone and what it is set at. Few vocalists will have much frequency content below 100 Hz, so this might be an appropriate setting (see Chapter 4, section The Microphone Preamp Stage) and will help to minimize potential sources of noise from mains hum or vibrations transferred to the microphone from the floor or microphone stand; however, leave this flat if there is any doubt.

In terms of positioning, a good guideline is to set the microphone so that is approximately a hand's span away from the vocalist at eye level, and a good microphone stand should always be used, even for the quickest of sessions. Position the microphone by booming it towards the vocalist from in front and slightly above, and at a little distance from him to keep it out of his way. However, the performer shouldn't sing/speak up to the microphone, but project straight ahead as he would in normal performance. Cables should be attached to the stand and kept well out of the way to avoid the microphone being pulled accidentally and to minimize trip hazards. If available, a suspension mounting should be used on the end of the stand, into which the microphone can be safely placed, avoiding possible vibrational disturbances from the stand or floor.

If the acoustics of the space allow it, a larger distance (up to a couple of feet) could be used. Remember the role proximity effect has when using some pressure difference microphones, and although appropriate for some vocal styles and performance preferences, it is not generally desirable in a studio recording. If for some reason close miking has to be used, employ the low-cut filter (at either microphone or mixing desk) to compensate for any increased bass end. The eye-height position serves two purposes. First, it will minimize the sound of breaths, pops, and other non-voiced utterances as the vocalist should be projecting past the microphone rather than onto it. Second, the human voice projects upper-mid frequencies (2–3 kHz)—those that carry the second formant and therefore maximize intelligibility of acoustic cues for most speech sounds, about 30 degrees upwards from the mouth (see Figure 3–3), and this position will help to accentuate this range.

Potential Problems

The most important problem to avoid with studio recording is that of "popping" distortion caused by plosive vocal sounds; hence, a pop shield should always be used in front of the microphone. A pop shield is a circular hoop covered in thin fabric mesh that acts to dissipate the acoustic pressure buildup caused by a plosive release, without affecting the overall sound. The foam windshields often supplied with microphones should not be used, as they tend to absorb higher frequencies. Professional pop shields can be expensive, but one can be easily made from some nylon stocking material stretched over a wire coat hanger or embroidery hoop. They are invaluable in studio vocal recording and should always be used. Problematic breath or vocal noises might also be an issue, but positioning the microphone as discussed above should help to minimize their effect—listen carefully when sound checking the vocalist for such noises and adjust positions accordingly, or advise as appropriate.

There is every chance that the performer will move around somewhat during the session, which can cause some problems with level settings at the desk/preamp. Although this can be compensated for to some extent by compression (see below) or changing the gain setting slightly as the session continues (often called "riding the fader"), it helps to get the performer to check his own positioning. To this end the pop shield can help again; place it where the vocalist is required to be, set the level for this position, and use the shield as a ref-erence point by asking the vocalist to ensure he sings up to it.

If neither positioning, pickup pattern, nor changing microphone acts to remove problematic sibilance, "de-essing" might be required (see below), but another handy trick is to place a pencil on the microphone grill, in the middle of the diaphragm, and hold it in place with a couple of elastic bands. A microphone with a flat frequency response will also help in this respect, rather than one with a presence peak. Finally, beware spill being picked up from the microphone originating from the vocalist's foldback headphones. This is especially the case if they aren't fully enclosed, or the singer has one ear off so that he can hear himself better. Generally, this won't be too much of a problem as it will be masked by other aspects of the final mix, unless of course the finished product has the vocalist performing unaccompanied for any length of time.

Effects Processing

In general, effects processing should not be used if at all possible when recording the voice in case they act to the detriment of the original signal or result in a final recording that cannot revert back to a raw and natural state. It is much better to add effects at the mixing/editing stage, as they can be applied nondestructively: any changes made can be undone to return to the original recording. However, in some cases, careful use of effects can enhance and help with the recording process, and the benefits of reverberation in the foldback mix has already been discussed above.

The most useful effect that can be applied when recording is compression. This will help to smooth out level changes caused by the vocalist moving around the microphone and ensure that signal peaks are controlled, minimizing the chance of clipping distortion. With careful setting of the compressor controls, it can act as an automatic "finger on the fader," adjusting the record level relative to the vocal signal level and responding much more quickly than an engineer acting to similar changes. However, care should be taken not to compress too much so that all dynamics are removed from the performance. A good starting point is to compress with a ratio of between 2:1 and 4:1, a very fast attack, and a release of about 0.5 s (or leave on auto), but with no more than 6 dB of gain reduction showing on the gain reduction meters. Note that riding the channel fader when recording may still be required to take care of large changes in signal level.

EQ can be used to tidy up the input signal and might be used in conjunction with low-cut filters to remove the very bottom end of the spectrum. However, it is best left flat to capture a natural and transparent performance. If for some reason the miked up sound is unsatisfac-

tory, changing microphone, pickup pattern, or position should be attempted first before resorting to EQ. It is always worthwhile spending more time at the recording stage to get the vocal sound right, rather than trying to correct the result with editing, mixing, or effects. Once safely recorded, EQ can be used in the post-recording stage for particular enhancements or to creative effect.

Gating can be used in extreme circumstances to avoid background or breath noise but must be carefully set up so as to not cut off the start or ends of phrases. Consider also that vocals with *no* breath noise sound unnatural. In general, however, this process is best applied post-recording.

If sibilance has proved to be a problem, *de-essing* is another useful post-recording process. A de-esser is a frequency dependent compressor that operates as shown in Figure 5–1. Essentially the side-chain now includes an additional EQ stage before the level detection stage. Note that a standard compressor can act as a de-esser by connecting a separate EQ to the side-chain

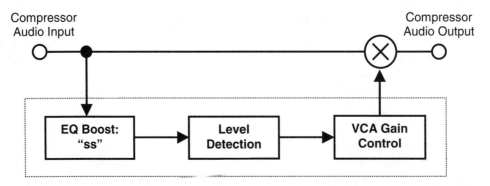

Figure 5–1. *The functional block diagram representation of a de-esser—a frequency dependent compressor. The side-chain now includes an EQ stage to boost the problematic sibilant frequencies. The result is that attenuation will only be applied to these aspects of the signal rather than the voice as a whole.*

input and decoupling the side chain from the audio input. In this case the input signal must be copied and routed in the mixing desk to two audio outputs —one for the compressor audio input and one for the EQ/compressor side-chain input. The EQ stage is designed to accentuate those problematic frequencies that are produced in sibilant speech/singing, typically in the 5–10 kHz region (see Figure 1–6 and Figure 2–19). As a result the compressor will only act on these aspects of the input signal and leave the rest untouched; sibilance on the audio input will be boosted in the side-chain, causing the signal level to pass the threshold setting and causing the level of the parallel audio signal to be reduced by the VCA gain control. The compressor controls will need to be set as usual, and again, subtle is better than dramatic for corrective processing. However, sibilance can also be used to good effect as the *ss* sounds can make vocal reverb sound bright and exciting over short passages. Apply slight cut at about or above 8 kHz if an actual de-esser is not used.

If working with a singer, double tracking the vocal line—getting him to sing the same part again—and mixing with the original can add depth, hide slight errors, and allow further creative possibilities. If this is not possible, or the two performances are too different, automatic double tracking (ADT) can be employed by running the original vocal line through a digital delay with a delay time of 15–35 ms (although up to 100 ms may work well). This delayed signal should then be modulated very slightly, using the delay modulation control (if this is an option) or either an additional *chorus* effect or pitch-shifting effect, with the latter set to detune the signal by

5–10 cents (100 cents = 1 semitone). The purpose of these effects is to add the very slight variations that will always be present in any two performances of the same vocal part. Again, subtlety is the key for a natural sound, and panning the two tracks left and right can add a further depth to the quality of the finished vocal. Reverberation can be very dramatic and effective when added to the spoken or singing voice at the mixing/editing stage. However, there is often a danger of putting too much reverb on the vocals because it usually sounds very good in isolation. In general, if the reverb on the vocals is noticeable when listening back to the mix, then it is probably too much.

Live Vocal Sound Reinforcement

In some aspects, recording a live vocal performance or working with a vocal in a sound reinforcement scenario is quite similar to what has preceded with studio recording. Certainly this is the case in terms of the source material, which will be solo male or female spoken or singing voice. However, both the location and the listening requirements are very different. The location will generally be a stage of some sort, which may be small or large, with an audience and sound mixing area somewhere in front and distinct from the stage area, and rather than transparent capture of the vocal source, the requirement is to project the performer across a wider area or audience. This voice source must compete with other instruments or performers in close proximity, some of which may be amplified or at significant acoustic level, and microphones will be working through a PA system with front-of-house and monitor speakers, all of which will conspire to cause problems with acoustic feedback. There may be restrictions in terms of microphone placement, and with such performances there is a one-and-only opportunity to get it right for the in situ audience—there is no second chance to correct errors as part of a later editing or mixing process. As with the studio, the performers are removed from the engineer, although this time by distance rather than solid barrier, and so effective communication must be established via the monitoring system when sound checking, and through visual cues during performance. Furthermore, any changes or corrections required to the sound once the performance has started are preferably corrected remotely from the FOH mixing desk position, rather than by having to go on-stage.

In terms of the listening environment, some of the possible problems have already been considered in Chapter 4, section Operational Guidelines, but the main purpose of this particular vocal application more than anything else is effective communication of performer vocal intent. As with studio recoding, the vocal line is usually the most important aspect of an ensemble performance and this must be delivered to the audience such that it can be understood clearly and easily above all other elements that the sound system is responsible for (or in terms of feedback, responsible for causing). This applies equally to spoken word, accompanied or unaccompanied singing, performance, or even the simplest voiceover announcements. However, it has to be accepted that, whereas in a studio environment there is usually the luxury of time, location, and equipment to get the best sound possible, generally being a transparent rendition of the vocal source, the

difficulties of live amplified performance impose a very particular set of restrictions, and compromises inevitably have to be made.

Microphone Choice and Positioning

The default microphone for live vocal work is a dynamic cardioid with a presence peak. Dynamic microphones are simple and rugged in terms of construction and therefore can be subjected to the rigors of repeated live performance work, where they may end up dropped or knocked through regular, repeated use or rigging/derigging as part of a longer tour. Noise floor levels are less critical for on-stage work, as there will be additional sources of possible noise from the PA, audience, other instruments, and performers that will potentially be more noticeable. Additionally, as they are less sensitive than condenser microphones, they are less susceptible to handling noise if the vocalist prefers not to use a stand.

The cardioid polar pattern will favor sounds from the front and is ideal for on-stage work, minimizing spill from other sound sources, with a null point at the rear ideal when a single monitor wedge speaker is used in front of the vocalist. A hypercardioid or supercardioid will give a little more "reach" due to their higher directivity index/distance factor (see Chapter 4, section on Microphone Directivity Patterns)—useful if the microphone is placed on a stand and the vocalist works a little way away from it (often found with backing vocalists), although the polar pickup pattern null point will change and hence monitor wedges should be placed off to one side accordingly (also discussed in Chapter 4, Operational Guidelines section). As these are all pressure difference microphones, they will all be subject to proximity effect. With studio recording, this was seen as a problem to be avoided through the use of low-cut filters or source distance, but in live work, the bass boost helps to reinforce the bottom end of the vocal, making it fuller and more powerful and helping it to cut through the overall mix. Similarly, the presence peak in the frequency response will help to provide clarity in the upper mid range, again helping the vocal to push above the background of any other instruments in the mix—although if the presence peak is too pronounced it may be a possible cause of feedback in the overall sound reinforcement system.

Unfortunately, there are few options in terms of microphone/source positioning, and the main requirement is feedback avoidance, so the main vocal microphone and stand should not be placed in front of the FOH speakers and should be positioned carefully in combination with vocalist position, monitor speaker positioning, and knowledge of the polar pickup null points. If the vocalist uses the microphone handheld for the majority of the time, he should be advised to use it close up to help minimize feedback, make best use of source level, and take advantage of the additional benefits provided by proximity effect. In some cases it may be more appropriate to consider using a headset microphone, usually with a wireless transmitter/receiver, to allow complete freedom of movement on stage; this is useful where a handheld microphone may detract from the performance (such as in musical theater). Such microphones will have a directivity pattern optimized for how they are used and worn, and this may include an omnidirectional polar response. Feedback may be a concern in such cases, although the close

proximity to the source, and the fact that they are usually condenser microphones, implies less gain applied at the mixing desk/preamp and hence the likelihood of this happening is somewhat reduced.

Potential Problems

The possibility of problematic feedback in such situations has been reiterated both here and in the previous chapter, and with some careful preparation, testing, and good microphone technique, its occurrence can be sufficiently minimized. There are a few additional problems that should also be considered, although there is little that can be done to avoid popping effects or breath noises/nonvocal utterances. The first problem comes from extraneous on-stage noise, including vibrations transferred to the microphone via the stand, handling noises, mains hum, etc. The easiest way to deal with such problems is to employ the low-cut filter on the mixing desk, or to cut using the low shelving EQ control. Both will help to generally tidy up the signal prior to its being further processed or amplified. The second possible problem is caused by spill from other instruments. For instance, in popular music it is very common to place the drum kit directly behind the singer, which means that some significant proportion of this signal will be picked up by the main vocal microphone. Again, microphone technique and performer positioning (if possible) might be able to help, as will any low cut applied to tidy up the bottom end. Similarly, a certain amount of attenuation in the high frequency shelving EQ band can help to some extent to minimize high frequency noise, for instance from cymbals. If applying corrective EQ in this manner, it is important to listen carefully to hear if it has any detrimental affect on the main vocal source.

Effects Processing

The use of EQ to tidy up the voice has been discussed above, and it is quick and easy to remove the very uppermost and lowermost frequencies with little implication for the actual source signal. Generally this is sufficient, unless there are significant vocal problems, such as a pronounced presence peak, leading to feedback (correct by applying narrow-band attenuation using a parametric EQ), or a general need for added vocal brightness (correct by applying a slight boost to the upper-mid frequency range). Gating can be very useful to help with problems of spill and to ensure a microphone is automatically turned off during times when the vocalist is not using it. It can also help to cut down on additional extraneous noise that might lead to possible feedback if the microphone is not being used in close. Again, the threshold must be set carefully to ensure all aspects of the performance are heard, especially the quieter sections, and attack and release controls should be checked so that the beginning and ends of words or phrases are not clipped off.

Compression should not be used; it may seem like a good idea to keep the vocal level consistent if the performer does not have the best microphone technique, but the compressor will also act to remove the dynamics from the performance. Perhaps even more importantly, as compression acts to boost the level of quieter signals, it can rapidly cause low level, potentially problematic, frequencies to be boosted into the danger region where feedback will rapidly occur. If level control is required, riding the fader may be sufficient or, alternatively, very slight compression with a high thresh-old and no makeup gain—essentially making the device act more as a limiter than a true compressor.

As for additional effects, reverb and delay can be applied as in studio applications. Delay in particular, if used subtly, can help to make the voice sound fuller and provide additional support during longer notes/passages. Although these effects can make the voice sound professionally produced and dramatic, if over-used or mixed too high they tend to clutter up the sound and hide the main direct sound—potentially leading to a lack of clarity, which is at odds with the main goal of live vocal sound reinforcement.

Spoken Word

Recording spoken word is not very different from general studio vocal work, although there are some additional issues that should be considered when preparing for a session. Sometimes these recordings can last over several days (for instance, when recording an audio book), and the key point to consider from the listener's perspective is consistency. Each session should have the same overall sound, and this should extend to sessions taking place after the main event that are used to take care of additional inserts, retakes, or edits. The final work will usually be selected from many different takes edited together, and so it is important that it seems like one smooth and continuous reading. If differences exist across edits they will sound very obvious and might result in many hours of additional painstaking editing and post-processing. Detailed note-taking is critical, and a digital camera can be very useful for taking snapshots of a particular setup for reference when replicating it at a later date. Issues to be aware of include signal level, microphone choice, placement, performer position, EQ, noise reduction or additional effects settings, the quality of the voice from day to day, and voice intonation due to position in the text.

Careful distancing of the performer is required, and the pop shield can again be used as a reference point, or a ruler (or similar item) can be used instead. If the recording is for dramatic production, beware of performer movement for a particular effect (e.g., walking away). Compensating with gain riding or compression might not be required, although clearly clipping will still need to be avoided. One significant difference with these sessions is that there is every possibility that the performer will be sitting down, often at a table, and he may have a script. The table will be a problematic source of reflections that will lead to possible phase cancellation and detrimental timbral coloration of the voice. The script may result in page-turning noises. Hence, careful microphone positioning together with sound checking is required, and so wherever possible, angle flat surfaces or microphones to minimize the chance of reflections bouncing right back into the microphone capsule. Music stands may prove useful for arranging pages or for providing a deflecting surface for reflections. Take time to get a good working setup and make note as to what it is for easy repeatability. Try to ensure the performer's head does not move too much during the recording or across sessions, as the directional property of the speech emanating from the mouth will lead to tonal imbalance; find a position the performer is comfortable with and a microphone position that works to best effect.

During the session the engineer should have his own copy of the written material on which to make edit notes, for instance where there are errors or where there are multiple takes. Rather than repeating a word that has been mispronounced or has a page turn alongside it, it is better to rerecord the whole sentence to ensure a smooth and easy edit post-recording.

DJs, either working in radio or providing mobile music services, might make use of a particular dynamics process called *ducking*. This is another variation on the compressor, as shown in Figure 5–2, although in this case the side-chain

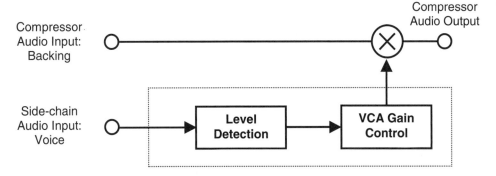

Figure 5–2. *The functional block diagram representation of a ducker. When a microphone is used, the voice signal routed to the side-chain input activates the compressor and causes any signal connected to the compressor input to be automatically attenuated, allowing the voice to come through clearly.*

input is decoupled from the actual audio input. The backing music acts as the compressor audio input, and the main vocal microphone signal is "copied" and routed in the mixing desk to an additional audio output that is connected to the compressor side-chain input. The compressor controls are set up as usual, with the result being that whenever the microphone is used, the additional signal level passes the side-chain threshold level and triggers the VCA to apply gain reduction to the audio signal passing through the regular audio input. This means that whenever the DJ speaks into the microphone, the music is automatically turned down so that he can be heard more clearly. When he stops talking, the backing music signal level will return to its original level according to the release time setting on the compressor.

Recording on Location

This section refers to recording the spoken voice out of doors and is important for film, television, and radio broadcast work, where the subjects may be actors, reporters, or interviewees. To a lesser extent it might also apply in some research contexts where recording must take place in nonstandard environments. Straight to camera television and radio reporting work are both relatively easy in this context as there is usually a single subject, and so one microphone can be used in close to record the speech. Film or television drama work can be much more involved and complicated, however. For a particular scene, good coverage will involve taking many shots from many different angles (wide, mid, close up, etc.), and so for the sound recordist this presents a wide variety of

material that must be captured cleanly and then later built into a believable audio world. Most importantly of all, when the camera changes angle, so will the sound, both in terms of listener perspective and the relative background noise. In this more complex recording environment, the goal is to capture the vocal performance of the actors as well and as cleanly as possible. This is made difficult by the fact, that although the camera might focus on a very small area, even the most directional of microphones will capture sound from the entire environment. Recording outside may remove the problem of troublesome reflections and reverberation (depending on location), but noise—and particularly environmental noise such as traffic, aircraft, wind, lighting hum, generators —becomes the major concern.

Microphone Choice and Positioning

In all such applications the vocal source(s) must be captured with the best clarity and quality of direct sound as possible, and so the best microphone for the conditions should be used. Outdoor work is often best recorded with a highly directional shotgun microphone (see Chapter 4, Microphone Directivity Patterns), although in a more enclosed environment it is less ideal as strong reflections or reverberation can act to color the timbre of the recorded voice. Shotguns should be used in combination with a shock mount to minimize handling noise, and it is imperative that even in the mildest conditions a professional windshield is used, as otherwise wind noise will add significant distortion to a vocal recording, be unpleasant for broadcast work, and render the source material unusable for film/TV production. Professional windshields are very noticeable as either large furry coverings or long plastic cylinders into which the microphone capsule is placed. Again, as was the case with studio microphones and vocal plosives, the foam coverings that microphones are supplied with do not provide sufficient protection and should not be relied upon in anything other than the mildest of conditions. In some cases, regular mono condenser microphones should be sufficient, especially if close up work is not required, and stereo-microphones (see Stereo Recording section) may also prove useful for the natural capture of the voice in a particular environment. However, for post-production work, where images and audio will be edited or creatively manipulated, having good quality direct sound is usually the best option, as background environmental noise can be added in separately. Small lavalier/lapel/tie-clip microphones can also work well as a primary or secondary backup method of capturing good quality direct sound, although in dramatic production it is clearly important that they and any cables are kept out of sight.

A shotgun microphone might be used with a pistol grip for working close to the source, but are more commonly used with a long "fish pole" boom arm, so that both microphone and sound recordist can be kept well clear of the camera shot. In both cases, it is important to maintain relative distance and orientation. Similarly, if the sources have to move, then the microphones will have to move around also, and so it is important to listen for timbral changes in the voice or obvious changes in background sound. In terms of background noise, as one would consider how to minimize the effect of possible problematic reflec-

tions when working indoors, it is worthwhile thinking how to best reject unwanted noise in favor of the direct sound through good position and microphone selection. If possible, adapt the acoustic environment, and if there is some trace of reverberation, try to minimize this as well, so that it can be added later and with more control in the post-production and editing process.

Potential Problems

As with recording spoken word in a studio environment, it is important to work with a script (if available) and make notes of problems, edits, takes, for later post-production editing. Although not critical in terms of general vocal production, in film/TV location work it is a good idea to record samples of general ambient sounds, noises, backgrounds in between dialogue shooting/recording, as this kind of material is invaluable in post-production to make the final result sound natural and believable, and it is used to bed in the vocals and other more specific sound effects. It can also be used to help mask problematic on-set sounds, such as lighting hum, that should not appear in the final production.

When transferring material into the digital audio workstation/editing workstation, it is important to carefully audition the recorded sound and make further notes as to what is usable or not, or what might require extensive editing or possible rerecording. It is therefore useful to keep recordings of all takes when on location, rather than just the final one, as earlier versions may have perfectly good audio that can be used to replace or correct problems with short passages of dialogue in an otherwise perfect final take. Listen out also for general noise, clipping, transients, and voice articulation problems, and when bedding in the dialogue track with more natural ambient background noise it is important to maintain and control level separation between the two for maximum flexibility in later editing stages. Errors in the dialogue track hidden in the background noise may become evident again if the voices need to be louder. If the dialogue needs to be quieter, the added background noise may become too loud and noticeable.

If there are severe problems with the voice recordings that cannot be corrected via editing, it must be recorded again. In film/TV production this is called *automatic dialogue replacement* (ADR; sometimes also called *post-synchro* or *looping*) and refers to the complete replacement of aspects of the dialogue elements by rerecording and looping with visual or audible feedback. It is an expensive process (in terms of actor time) and therefore budget vs. quality issues might define the final outcome; every effort should be made to fix the problem via editing wherever possible. When carrying this out remember what microphones were used at the original recording stage and use them again wherever possible. It might even help to use more than one of the same microphone positioned to match sound changes due to different shots used in the original production sound. All this is done to ensure that the same overall vocal timbre is maintained across edits and may even extend to using the same windshield if it acts to color the sound in any way. It is also useful to have the original production sound available as a reference for both the engineer and the actor. ADR will take place in a typical studio or screening environment, and hence the same guidelines as appropriate for studio recording work will apply.

Effects Processing

The most important thing to consider in terms of effects when location recording is that there is very little option for using them, given the limitations of both portability and the possible lack of mains power. Some portable digital recorders may include a built-in limiter or compressor to help minimize the chance of clipping, but these may not be as reliable or as good quality as more comprehensive studio devices. The main thing to consider here is that effects will be limited to post-production only, demanding good use of headroom and level control when in the field.

Anechoic Recording

The final consideration for solo voice recording is the possible use of an anechoic chamber as the location. These are special rooms designed to be acoustically isolated from their surroundings, to have a very low noise floor, and most importantly of all, to be essentially reflection free. Reflections, and therefore also reverberation, are eliminated through the use of alternately arranged foam wedges across walls, ceiling, and floor. The latter point implies that the "working" floor is actually suspended above the real, acoustically absorbing floor and is accomplished by being constructed from a strong metal grill. An example of what the walls in an anechoic chamber look like is shown in Figure 5–3.

Hence, anechoic chambers present an optimal environment for high quality recording work where a direct sound only, dry voice source is required, and they are commonly used in research applications where critical acoustic measurements or recordings are made.

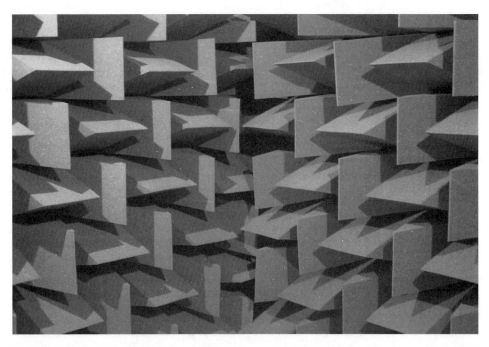

Figure 5–3. *The walls in an anechoic chamber. The foam wedges are designed and arranged to absorb virtually all incident sound resulting in a reflection-free, and hence reverberation-free, environment. This, together with excellent acoustic isolation and a low noise floor, makes it an ideal recording space for critical work.*

The low noise floor and acoustic isolation also help in this respect, but perhaps most important of all in terms of vocal recording is the fact that a reflection-free environment implies that high quality, flat frequency, omnidirectional microphones can be easily used without the usual additional concerns relating to positioning, background noise, and reverberation. Anechoic chambers are also useful in more commercial work where high quality reverberation or spatialization is required as part of the mixing/editing process, where the source recordings need to be as dry as possible in order to achieve the best effect. However, accessibility to these chambers and the expense in building or hiring them usually prohibits their common use in such projects.

There are two problems to be aware of when recording in such an environment. The first is to consider any equipment that is brought into the space along with the vocal performer, as it is very likely that there will be no readily available audio connections to a remotely placed control room as in a normal studio. It is very common to use a modern laptop computer and audio hardware/software combination to do the recording as this is a powerful, flexible, and portable combination. However, cooling fans used internally to keep the computer cool will be a possible source of additional noise that will be very evident in an otherwise very quiet environment. Sometimes these fans might not be activated until some time into the recording session after the computer has been working hard for some time. Computer hard drives can also be sources of noise. In such a situation it is very worthwhile to try to source quiet equipment that will not cause such problems. Non-computer based stand-alone recorders or flash memory devices that have no mechanical parts might be good compromises. Alternatively, arrange additional absorbing material around the noisy equipment and place it carefully away from the vocal source in a corner of the chamber if possible. The other consideration with bringing in additional equipment is that it may be a possible cause of acoustic reflections (e.g., a laptop screen), and so careful positioning and the use of additional absorbing material should be considered.

The second problem to consider is the nature of the environment itself and its impact on the vocal performer. Listening to one's own voice in a completely reflection-free environment is a very unusual experience and can become tiring after prolonged exposure. Regular rest breaks in the session might be required, or alternatively, the performer should have a good headphone foldback mix with some additional reverberation added. If the latter approach is used, care should be taken to keep levels low to avoid headphone sound leaking into the microphone.

MULTIPLE VOCAL SOURCES

Introduction

Whereas the entire purpose of the previous section was to use microphone and recording techniques to remove the solo vocal source from the surrounding environment, this section is concerned with capturing the entire acoustic event—the sound of the voice source in the acoustic space within which it has been placed. Generally, this implies that there is no longer a solo performer but rather a number of vocalists that make up the specific sonic event. These vocalists may be spatially distinct and therefore considered as separate solo sources or, more commonly, be grouped together in an ensemble such as a choir. Stereo microphone techniques are also introduced as these methods are generally more appropriate for capturing the complete source plus environment combination rather than just the individual source. The one exception to this that was not included in the previous section is soloist recording in a performance venue without sound reinforcement. In this scenario, the desire is again to capture the sound of the complete event rather than the individual, and a stereo recording is the most appropriate solution. Hence, this special case is covered as part of what follows.

Stereo Recording

Under normal listening conditions we use our two ears, separated by our head, to locate the direction from which a sound source is originating. We rely on a number of auditory mechanisms to help us determine this source direction and they are summarized as follows.

Interaural Time Difference (ITD)

Depending on direction, the sound source will arrive at one ear before the other, resulting in a very small amount of difference in arrival time between left and right ears. This only works for low frequencies.

Interaural Level Difference (ILD)

Depending on direction, the sound source will be louder in the ear that is oriented more closely to the source, resulting in level difference between left and right ears of up to 20 dB SPL at some frequencies. This does not work at low frequencies, as the sound wave will diffract around the head such that the level difference between the two ears is negligible.

Pinnae Cues

ITD and ILD only give enough information to locate a source in two dimensions. The actual shape of the outer ear imparts a direction dependent frequency characteristic on the incident sound that helps to resolve front-back and up-down differences.

Head Movement

When attempting to work out the direction of a sound source, very slight head movements act to constantly change the relative ITD, ILD, and pinnae cues so that a listener can more easily and quickly determine source location. Primarily this acts to minimize ITD and ILD values to a point that they are essentially zero. This implies that the sound source is either directly in front of or behind the listener, and pinnae cues—and of course sight—can help to determine the final source direction.

With knowledge of these directional properties of the ear, particularly those relating to ITD and ILD, it is possible to fool the ear into perceiving a directional effect through just a pair of speakers or headphones—what we typically refer to as *stereophonic* or *stereo* audio presentation. There are two main ways of recording stereo sound images for presentation over a pair of loudspeakers—*coincident stereo* and *spaced stereo* microphone techniques.

Coincident Stereo Microphone Recording

This technique uses a pair of identical directional (not omnidirectional) microphones, each connected to a separate audio channel. To create robust, stable sound images suitable for stereo presentation, it is considered important to minimize time differences between left and right channels, and so the two microphones must be placed as close together as is physically possible—hence the term coincident stereo (also known as, XY, crossed pair, or normal stereo). The result is that sound sources are captured with differing levels between the two channels. This is due to the directional characteristics of the microphones used and the fact that signal amplitudes will vary in direct relation to the physical angle between the microphone pair and the sound source. Hence, this technique works well at presenting realistic and natural stereo sound because it is based on how the ILD works with the auditory system. The normal method is to place the capsule of one microphone immediately above the other, so that they are coincident in the horizontal plane, which is the dimension from which sound image positions will be created.

Coincident stereo is actually based on simple amplitude panning, as implemented in the mixing desk channel pan control (see Chapter 4, Routing and Output section), where altering the relative level of a mono signal between two stereo speakers will cause the sound image to be perceived as moving between them. This same relative panning effect can be replicated for a sound source moving between two coincident figure-of-eight microphones at an angle of 90 degrees to each other. This arrangement of microphones is called a *Blumlein pair*, after Alan Blumlein, who first experimented with these techniques in the 1930s, and the resultant polar pickup patterns are shown in Figure 5–4.

The Blumlein pair arrangement gives accurate stereo imaging between two loudspeakers of the original position of the acoustic source. Note that the stereo image will be reversed for sources to the rear. Ideally, the 90 degree angle should be maintained and all relevant sources should be within the *acceptance angle*; this is defined as the usable working area in front of the microphone as defined by their polar patterns, and as also used when considering single microphones, as already discussed in the section Microphone Directivity Patterns in Chapter 4. Acceptance angle will therefore act to restrict the range of possible source to

microphone distances that will result in good stereo playback. The acceptance angle for a Blumlein pair is 70 degrees.

If cardioid microphones rather than figure-of-eights are used, the angle between the capsules needs to be wider in order to produce the same relative level differences between microphones for a given source position. This angle is actually taken as the point at which the response drops by 3 dB relative to the on-axis position, and for cardioids is defined as 131 degrees, as shown in Figure 5–5. This gives a much wider acceptance angle of 130 degrees, meaning that the pair can be moved closer to the source.

In practice, 90 degrees (giving an acceptance angle of 170 degrees) is the commonly used angle of separation for a crossed pair of cardioids, as it is easiest to set up, although it is possible to change this angle over a small range to

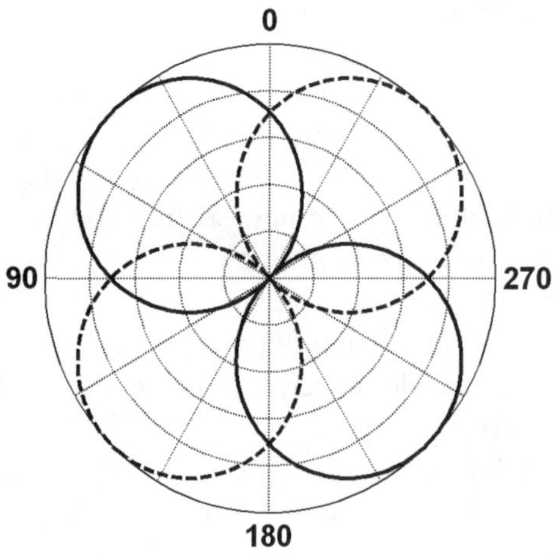

Figure 5–4. *The directivity patterns of a crossed pair of figure-of-eight microphones, used for coincident stereo recording. The angle of separation is 90 degrees, and this is also known as a Blumlein pair. This arrangement will result in the same stereo imaging as a standard mixing desk channel pan pot.*

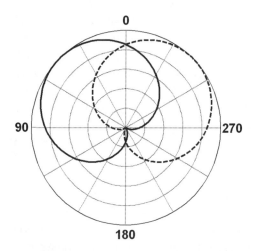

Figure 5–5. *The directivity patterns of a crossed pair of cardioid microphones, used for coincident stereo recording. The angle of separation for level differences equivalent to a Blumlein pair is 131 degrees.*

adjust the precise relationship between the physical sound source positions in front of the microphones and their perceived positions in the stereo image. Greater than 130 degrees will leave a "hole-in-the-middle" of the stereo field where there will be a noticeable drop in level and where central sound sources will fall outside the optimal polar pickup angle of each microphone. If the angle is smaller than 80 degrees, the acceptance angle becomes greater than 180 degrees, with the small focused overlap of the microphone directivity patterns meaning that lateral sound sources are considerably attenuated. A coincident pair based on hypercardioid microphones will be halfway between a cardioid and figure-of-eight, and hence the angle between the capsules should be 105 degrees.

One problem with the crossed pair techniques is that the center of the vocal source is off-axis from both microphones. This can lead to timbral coloration due to the less-than-ideal off-axis frequency response of the microphones. *Mid-side* (M-S) recording uses one microphone to capture the *middle* signal, which would be obtained if the outputs of a stereo crossed pair were added together. The other microphone captures the *side* signal, which would be obtained if the output of one microphone was subtracted from the other. The most common arrangement is to use a cardioid microphone facing forward (the mid microphone) together with a figure-of-eight microphone (the side microphone) facing sideways at 90 degrees, as shown in Figure 5–6. When these M-S signals are converted into normal left-right stereo, they produce an identical acceptance angle to conventional crossed cardioids.

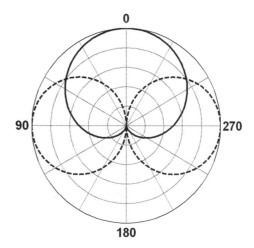

Figure 5–6. *The directivity patterns of a mid-side coincident microphone arrangement. The mid microphone is a cardioid that will be on-axis with the source (rather than off-axis with a crossed pair). The side microphone is a figure-of-eight. After conversion to normal stereo, this arrangement allows manipulation of the stereo image acceptance angle and to some extent the balance of direct to reflected sound.*

The two signals have to go through a conversion process before being auditioned on loudspeakers or headphones as in normal left-right stereo. The most useful aspect of the system for everyday recording tasks is that the acceptance angle and hence the perceived spread of sound sources across the stereo image can be controlled easily from the mixing desk or even after the recording. This will also to some extent allow control over the direct to lateral sound—giving some control over the amount of reverberation received relative to the direct sound. As the level of the mid microphone is increased relative to the side microphone, the useful acceptance angle and hence the perceived width of the stereo field is increased. As the level of the mid microphone decreases the acceptance angle and relative stereo field also decreases. The M-S signals are converted to conventional stereo as follows:

1. Pan the M microphone to the center.
2. Split the S microphone to feed a pair of adjacent channels.
3. Pan the S channels hard left and right, phase reversing the right channel.
4. Listen with the monitoring switched to mono and balance the gains of the two S channels for minimal output.
5. Revert to stereo monitoring, and fade up the M channel.
6. Adjust the balance between the M and S signals for the desired image spread.

Note that it is also possible to use specific stereo microphones consisting of multiple microphone diaphragms in a single capsule, which makes the process of setting up for a stereo recording session significantly easier. In some stereo microphone designs the internal arrangement is fixed, in others it is variable and some control over the stereo image will be facilitated through external controls. Designs exist based on both the crossed pair technique and the M-S arrangement, with the latter giving somewhat greater flexibility for stereo field manipulation as part of the post-recording editing/mixing process.

Spaced Microphone Techniques

This method uses two (or more) identical but spaced microphones, each connected to a separate audio channel as before. However, with this technique, as the microphones are spatially separated,

a sound will arrive at each capsule at a slightly different time according to the relative distance between it and the source. Hence, the spaced microphones effectively receive time-of-arrival information, and so this technique generates a stereo image based on timing differences (rather than level differences) and is comparable to how ITD works with the auditory system. However, the final stereo image, when presented over loudspeakers, is less stable and robust when compared with a similar coincident recording. This is because the sound emanating from each loudspeaker will arrive at both left and right ears (rather than left speaker to left ear only, right speaker to right ear only), and there will be a slight time delay added to the additional signal received at the opposite ear due to the off-center positioning of each speaker, as shown in Figure 5–7. This additional set of ITDs imparted onto the ITDs of the original spaced microphone recording tends to lead to confusion in terms of where a source is perceived to originate from.

An additional disadvantage—although less critical in modern audio distribution—is that if the outputs from the spaced microphones are mixed together to produce a single mono signal, the timbre of the overall mix might be altered due to phase cancellation effects (compare with problematic reflections when miking a single source and how direct and reflected path can cause the same effects). The greater the number of combined microphones, the worse the effect is likely to be. The big advantage of spaced miking, however, is that this technique allows the use of omnidirectional microphones, as the relative level of the acoustic source and how it varies with direction is not critical. The implication

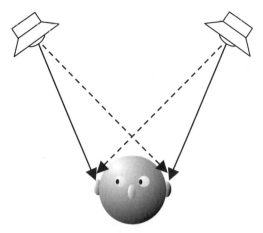

Figure 5–7. *When listening to stereo material using two loudspeakers, an additional set of interaural time difference auditory cues will be imparted onto the audio signal. This is due to the fact that the signal from each loudspeaker will arrive at both ears, and in each case the dotted line path is slightly longer than the solid line path, implying a time-of-arrival difference. This can confuse stereo information that is already dependent upon time differences captured from spatially separate microphones, leading to poor stereo imaging.*

of using such microphones is a significantly improved frequency response, particularly in the low end, and a more natural and transparent sound.

Although not necessarily accurate or stable in terms of stereo imaging, the final sound is normally perceived as having width and a certain amount of imaging information, and it usually sounds more spacious than a coincident recording. The recording might also suffer from a hole-in-the-middle if the microphones are too widely spaced apart. The simplest spaced microphone technique is to place an identical pair of omnidirectional microphones a distance apart in front of the sound source. A microphone spacing of between about a half and a

third of the width of the actual sound stage [the width of the source(s) that must be recorded] is a good place to start in terms of positioning. This could be improved through the use of additional directional microphones to alleviate any potential hole-in-the-middle effects. Other spaced techniques that use directional microphones are often called *near coincident* techniques because they combine the level difference recording characteristics of directional coincident microphones with spaced arrays. For instance, the *ORTF* method uses a pair of cardioid microphones with a separation angle of 110 degrees spaced about 17 cm apart from one another.

Multiple Soloists

Working with multiple soloists is based on an extension of the techniques introduced in the section, Single Vocal Sources, when recording the solo voice. As with the other applications discussed so far, the final listeners should be first considered when approaching the problem—what perspective will they have on the presented sound, and what is important for them to hear? If the multiple voices are supposed to be heard in the context of the space in which they are presented, it is probably best to consider them as an ensemble and to use a stereo recording technique to capture the sound of the overall event (see the section, Ensemble Recording). However, this will generally only apply to a limited set of possible applications, such as classical-style music performance, and there are a great many other situations where clarity of direct sound, separation, and control are more important factors to be considered. Examples might include studio recording of multiple lead vocal lines, sound reinforcement of lead and backing vocals in amplified performance, interviews for radio or television broadcast, musical theater, and even applications such as teleconferencing. In each case, once the individual vocal sources are captured they will be subject to further manipulation, editing, or studio processing post-capture.

Sources and Location

In terms of location, studio work is generally the easiest to control as there should be enough space to separate the vocal performers, and this can be improved through the use of acoustic screens. Generally, the acoustics of a studio space will not influence the final recording too much, particularly if care is given to source and microphone positioning, and this will of course be helped further by using directional microphones. The main problem to consider will be spill from each performer bleeding into the other microphones, so achieving good sound source separation is important. However, problematic spill may well be masked when placed in the context of the wider music production and so might not be too serious a problem, although every effort should be made to minimize its effects. Working with multiple solo performers in an anechoic environment will offer many of the advantages of the studio in terms of control and clarity of direct sound. Care should be given to the possibility of problematic reflections, however, and there might not be as much space available in which to arrange the vocalists themselves. Studio based radio broadcasting will be a very similar situation given that the environment is optimized for the best sound for spoken voice, with good separation between announcers/ broadcasters, and little influence from the surrounding acoustics.

Just about every other example of working with multiple vocal performers will introduce problems related to the recording environment that will have to be considered and solved. Live sound reinforcement work is a simple extension of the solo vocalist case, although with every additional performer and microphone used will come the requirement for additional foldback monitoring and therefore another potential source of feedback. Every separate channel of monitoring should have a dedicated pre-fade auxiliary send from the main FOH mixing desk (if a separate monitoring desk is not being used) and most importantly its own graphic EQ for tuning out problematic frequencies. These vary with positioning and source-microphone distance, and so each microphone/monitor combination will require its own individual EQ settings. Also the more microphones that are used on stage, the more spill picked up from other off-axis sources. Therefore, non-critical microphone channels should be muted when not in use, or noise gates used to achieve the same effect automatically. Again, this will help to minimize possible feedback and generally make the mixing process easier. Obviously, directional microphones should be used at all times.

Other forms of broadcasting, particularly those based in television studios, will make use of lavalier/lapel/tie-clip microphones to ensure good capture of direct sound from each individual. Care should be taken in positioning the microphone well. The "tie" position works best, as it will center the microphone with the mouth, although it should not be so high that the chin shadows the microphone, perhaps when the person's head moves to read written notes. Generally, such microphones also have a rolled off bass-response to take care of possible proximity effects if it has a cardioid family directivity pattern, and to compensate for a possible bass-rise from the resonance of the person's chest cavity. Similarly, the high end may be boosted slightly to compensate for the microphone being positioned off-axis. In general, once attached, the resulting sound should be checked for any major problems or variability as the talker goes about his regular business. This should include checking that the microphone sound/positioning is not affected by the subject's normal movements.

These types of microphones, usually mounted in a headset, are also used extensively in theater productions (especially musical theater) where the challenge is to get good sound from each actor while keeping the microphone and cables out of sight as much as possible. They are often only used for the principal performers, and so for capturing, for instance, the chorus or other on-stage sound, shotgun microphones are arranged around the edge of the stage to give good overall coverage. Graphic EQ might again have to be used to minimize feedback, although the levels involved are generally considerably less than amplified sound reinforcement and so are less of a problem. Another type of microphone used in this and similar vocal applications is the *boundary microphone*—sometimes also called a *float*. These microphones generally have a hemispherical (half omnidirectional) pickup pattern and are designed to be mounted on a flat surface (such as the front stage area or a wall). They operate on a different principle from the micro-

phones introduced so far (although they are generally a condenser type design) and use the acoustics of direct and reflected sound at a surface to give effective rejection of nondirect/reflected sound in favor of direct sound only (and hence will also help to minimize feedback problems). However, despite their good rejection of background sound, given their almost omnidirectional behavior, they should be used with care in terms of source pickup, applied gain, and possible feedback. Also, as they have to be physically placed on a wall or floor, they will be subject to possible mechanical vibrations from, for instance, footsteps.

In research applications, if multiple talkers or singers must be captured simultaneously, with clarity, separation, and accuracy being the important influencing factors, probably the only option available is to use headset microphones. If the recording location is large, with a controlled acoustic such that good separation can be achieved and reflections and spill minimized, there may be more options available, and the use of spaced omnidirectional microphones (favored for research applications) might be possible. However, this is generally unlikely given that the favored space for this approach would be a large anechoic chamber. Generally then, the headset method is perhaps the best way forward and has been reported as being successful in a number of studies. Note that additional microphones may be required to ensure that the headset microphones are calibrated correctly, as detailed in the section Recording for Research.

Where there is a requirement to capture multiple talkers and individual lavalier/headset microphones are not practical or possible, a simple one-to-one arrangement of spaced directional microphones is probably the best option. This may be used for instance in round-table style conference presentations, or in multiple talker teleconferencing. In the latter application, if source separation is not critical a single (for mono) or multiply arranged (for stereo) boundary microphones placed appropriately will provide a good compromise. As with theater sound, care should be taken to avoid possible sources of mechanical vibrations that will be captured due to the microphone being directly placed on a local surface—typically a tabletop in this case—with drumming fingers or moving papers, pens, etc., being obvious sources.

Potential Problems

In the majority of these applications, the purpose of the sound system used is to ensure that the direct sound is captured in such a way that is it clear and separate from background sounds, particularly the other sources present in the local vicinity, so that control can be obtained over each individual source. However, as soon as more that one microphone is used—for even a single source—then the application verges on being a spaced stereo recording, even if single channel capture is the required outcome. This means that the related problems already discussed in this and the previous chapter are combined and must be considered and dealt with. These can be summarized as follows.

Omnidirectional vs. cardioid family. Omnis will give a flat frequency response and transparent sound at the expense of loss of separation and increased spill and background sound (including reverberation and reflections). Cardioid family microphones will improve separation and reject nondirect sound but poten-

tially alter the timbre of the captured vocal source.

Source separation and background noise. Priority is given to the capture of the individual direct voice source and rejection of background noise to facilitate maximum control of individual sources. However, no microphone is ideal, and every microphone added to a particular scenario will capture every source present to some degree, reducing separation and ultimately compromising control.

Off-axis colorization. Nondirect sounds will be captured off-axis by other nearby microphones. The off-axis frequency response of a directional microphone is not at all ideal, leading to potential timbral colorization problems when multiple channels are summed or auditioned together—giving a total result that consists of optimal on-axis direct sound from the source microphone, together with colored, off-axis spill captured from another adjacent microphone.

Phase cancellation effects. Spaced microphones imply captured timing differences for a particular source. This may lead to phase cancellation based timbral colorization due to the delay between signals when summed or auditioned together and/or confused stereo imaging. This problem will be more pronounced if there are major reflections also present.

As a helpful guideline, wherever possible, aim to have the distance between spaced microphones at least three (and preferably closer to five) times that of the individual source-microphone distance. In summary, maintaining good separation is the key to achieving a good recording or good sound in these and other similar multiple solo source scenarios. Time, experimentation, and positioning will all help in this regard and ultimately provide greater flexibility, control, and creative options in editing, mixing, and post-production stages.

Ensemble Recording

Ensemble recording here refers to the capture of vocalists performing in a particular venue. Source separation is not the key focus; rather, priority is given to the accurate and transparent capture of the whole sound event, to include all performers, their relative balance, blend, and spatial positioning, and the acoustics of the venue itself. The most common example of where these techniques are appropriate would be choral recording, although this may include much smaller ensembles such as a barbershop quartet or the performance of spoken word. Note, however, that with smaller ensembles, production or aesthetic preferences may dictate that they should be recorded as multiple individual sources, as discussed in the previous section, rather than as a natural whole ensemble. Sound reinforcement is less common, as ensembles are sized for the material and space in which they will be heard, although individual microphones may be used to help soloists as part of the wider group (for instance spoken narration plus choral performance), and the use of such *spot microphones* will be considered as part of this section. In this context, the ensemble considered will also include solo performers where individual close-up miking is less appropriate and the sound in its totality in combination with the space is the desired result. Ultimately, what is being attempted is the capture and permanent recording of a particular sonic event so that the listener hears what the audience would have heard in the venue (often in the best seat) during the performance itself. Hence, stereo microphone techniques are the primary method of realizing this desire.

Source and Location

In general, the aim is to arrange the ensemble around the stereo microphone arrangement in such a way that they occupy the complete stereo image, or rather to place the microphones so that they capture the complete stereo sound stage. Considering a large choir, as might be found accompanying an orchestra, as the vocal ensemble source, coincident crossed cardioids might be best placed above and close to the conductor position in order to achieve the desired stereo image width. However, a Blumlein pair of crossed figure-of-eights would have to be positioned a long way down the venue, much further away from the choir, to achieve the same stereo width due to their narrower acceptance angle of 70 degrees. In choosing the polar patterns for the stereo microphone arrangement, the physical separation between sound sources and microphones is determined for a given stereo width and therefore the listener's perspective of the recording.

In this example the cardioids would give a very close-perspective sound, with little reverberation, due to both close positioning and directivity pattern influenced rear rejection, and a distorted choral balance favoring those singers closer to the front and more centrally positioned. The figure-of-eights would give a much more natural and balanced perspective to the choir, but would also capture a great deal of the reverberant sound, due to both their positioning and their increased rear pickup, which might make the recording rather more distant than anticipated. A compromise solution might use crossed hypercardioid mikes at some midpoint between cardioid and figure-of-eight extremes, or a scattering of close spot microphones to reinforce the weaker sections of the choir.

Microphone Positioning

As a starting point, the most commonly used method and easiest to get good results while still allowing a degree of experimentation is the crossed pair. These should be good quality cardioid condenser microphones, positioned one above the other, angled at between 90 and 120 degrees, according to source width. As mentioned above, they will also help to cut down on the amount of reverberation captured in the recording, due to the null pickup point at their rear. In general, a good level of direct sound compared with the reverberant sound is required to ensure overall clarity. Placing the microphones in a typical audience seat location will usually result in too much reverb when auditioned over loudspeakers. Experiment with distance to achieve the best balance between closeness/clarity and liveness/reverberance. It helps when setting source-microphone distance to have an estimate of the critical distance/reverberation radius of the space where direct and reverberant sound for a particular source are theoretically balanced. Clearly, the microphones should not be placed beyond this distance. It obviously helps when experimenting with position in this way to be able to listen directly to the results from the microphones to aid the decision-making process. If possible, stereo loudspeakers in a separate control room should be used, although realistically for most scenarios, good headphone (preferably enclosed) listening will be the main method of monitoring the microphone signals.

Once an optimum distance for the microphones has been decided the stereo imaging produced by the coincident pair should be considered. Monitor the performers over headphones and listen to make sure that what is heard agrees with what can be seen and heard in the actual venue. If the stereo spread is either too wide or too narrow, then the angle of separation (and hence the acceptance angle) can be adjusted. If the stereo image appears off-center, ensure that gain levels are equal for both microphone channels and that they are pointing in the appropriate direction. If possible, before the performers enter the venue, make a recording of someone walking across the front of the performance area from stage left to stage right and listen back to the result to make sure the recorded stereo imaging is in good agreement.

Always use stands that give good stability and allow the microphones to be raised to a good, high level. Raising or lowering the microphones in this manner can also achieve a good balance between any soloists and the accompanying ensemble if this is required, or the ensemble as a whole if it consists of many people. Use shock mounts wherever possible to minimize possible noise from vibrations, or place the stands on some rubber or sponge mats to decouple them from the floor of the venue (carpet tiles can also be useful). A good starting position in terms of microphone distance and height is about 12 feet from the performers and about 12 feet above the floor.

Potential Problems

If it is not possible to achieve an optimum balance between direct and reflected sound or stereo width due to limitations of time in setting up or restrictions in terms of microphone positioning, a combination technique might have to be used. This consists of a main stereo pair together with individual spot microphones. This technique is also appropriate if additional minimal sound reinforcement is required for particular aspects of the ensemble or for soloists working with them in combination, or if an omnidirectional spaced pair is used as the main microphone arrangement resulting in a hole-in-the-middle stereo imaging problem. A spot microphone is basically a close-up microphone used in combination with a more distanced main stereo pair to reinforce or generally improve the overall balance of sound sources. There are three things to consider with this combination technique.

Image position. The main microphone pair will establish stereo image positions for each aspect of the ensemble, and the close-up spot microphones should not contradict this virtual sound stage. Hence, each spot microphone must be panned appropriately to match the main stereo mix. The best technique for setting the individual pan positions is to concentrate on the stereo image of a particular vocal part from the main stereo pair, then slowly fade up the corresponding spot microphone, paying particular attention to how the image moves in the stereo field as this happens. If the image

pulls to the right, fade the spot microphone down, adjust the pan control slightly more to the left, and try again. Repeat until the pan position of the spot microphone is in agreement with the main stereo pair.

Perspective. A microphone close to the vocal source will have a completely different perspective to one much further away. This contrast is usually undesirable as it will draw undue attention to the soloist in question. The relative balance between the direct sound from the spot microphone and the overall direct-plus-reverberation mix from the main pair is critical. If the signal from the spot microphone is too noticeable then it is too high in the overall mix.

Timing. Note that this is usually only a problem with very large recording venues. Consider again the recording of a large choir in a large venue where the main stereo microphones may be 50 feet away from the main ensemble. Sound travels at approximately one foot per millisecond (ms), and so the signal from the stereo pair will be delayed by about 50 ms relative to any close spot microphones. Therefore, to ensure that close-up and distant microphones are in agreement, the spot microphones must be delayed by the appropriate amount, usually at the editing or mixing stage. It is therefore important in this case to measure source-microphone distances, and if appropriate, the temperature of the venue, which will help to give a good estimate of the speed of sound. From this a time delay can be calculated, with final adjustments made by ear to suit (see Chapter 1, section Sound Transmission and Velocity, and some of the suggested further reading for more information relating to how the speed of sound varies with temperature and how this calculation would be performed).

Finally, if the stereo pair used, for whatever reason, tends to favor the direct sound from the ensemble, resulting in a slightly too close perspective, some additional control over the reverberation can be facilitated through the use of two additional spaced "ambient" microphones. These microphones should be placed beyond the critical distance of the space, with generally a spaced arrangement giving better results than a similar coincident pair, and they are used to capture the more reverberant sound of the venue. Once in place, they should be balanced up with the more direct coincident pair to give more control over direct/reverberant perspective of the finished result. However, both this and spot miking methods do add to the complexity of the overall recording (a mixing desk or multitrack recording system will be required rather than a two-track direct to stereo device), and so it is usually best to experiment with the main stereo pair to get the best sound, balance, and perspective that is possible for a particular source/location/listener combination.

Background Vocals in Popular Music

Background vocals in studio recording work are sometimes dealt with somewhat differently from what has been considered so far and are therefore considered separately here. Note that background vocals in amplified sound reinforcement applications should be treated as individual soloists for clarity, separation,

control, and minimization of feedback. This may also apply in the studio according to production or aesthetic considerations. However, it is generally assumed that in studio work there will be adequate control over the acoustics of the actual recording space and so a little more flexibility is allowed.

General background vocals (sometimes called "gang" vocals) involve grouping a number of performers around a single microphone rather than miking individually. This helps to provide a uniformity of sound, will give a particular energy to the recorded music, and allows the vocalists to interact with one another for the sake of the overall performance. A cardioid microphone, preferably a condenser, can be used for this, but the limitations of the acceptance angle and the possibility of off-axis colorization should be considered. As a result, there should be no more than two or three vocalists grouped in an arc around the front of the microphone. If the acoustics of the studio environment allow it, an omnidirectional directivity pattern would be ideal, providing a more transparent sound and allowing many more vocalists to be arranged around the microphone in a circle at an equal distance. As with stereo recording, the source-microphone distance in either configuration will alter the overall sense of perspective of the ensemble when auditioned.

If further stereo control is required to further enhance the overall production, it is relatively simple to replace the cardioid/omni with a coincident pair. The next level of improved separation and control would be to record each vocalist individually and at the same time. In this situation hypercardioid microphones will help to focus in on each individual performer, and acoustic screens should be used if available. As with any technique involving multiple spaced microphones, the possibility of spill and phase cancellation effects should be considered, but this will allow individual panning of each source while helping to maintain the group vocal feel. Of course, the final level of control would be to record each vocalist separately and deal with them as any other solo vocal performer.

SUMMARY

This chapter has considered a wide variety of vocal recording and sound reinforcement applications and how they should be approached to achieve the best results. The definition of what might be "best" varies from case to case but should similarly be defined on a case-by-case basis through due consideration of the nature of the sound source, the environment in which it is being recorded, and perhaps most importantly of all, the demands or reasoning behind the final listening experience. There are many different scenarios where a vocalist has to work with a microphone and associated audio system, and a distinction has been made between single or multiple vocal sources. The particular demands of recording for vocal research have also been considered. Single source work introduces the importance of capturing the direct sound from the source while minimizing spill, background noise, reverberation, and/or feedback, with the implication this has for clarity, separation, and control over the final result. Ensemble vocal work introduces the use of stereo recording techniques and the importance of recording a complete

sound event in such a way that what the final listeners hear is a true representation of what they would have heard had they sat in the best seat in the house during the event. It should also be clear that this is a somewhat artificial delineation, as there are some scenarios that fall into both camps—for instance, recording a solo singer in a good concert hall.

It is important to note that the contents of this chapter should be considered as guidelines, rather than rules. Generally, there are no hard and fast rules when it comes to recording—the ultimate deciding factor is that the final result should sound "good." Again, the definition of *good* is highly subjective and will also vary according to the particular recording task. Making quality recordings for research purposes is a particular example here, although objective measures can also be applied to some extent in this case to determine the final quality of the results obtained. Some of the most important points to take away from this chapter actually have nothing to do with microphones and audio systems at all, but have everything to do with being a good sound engineer:

- Plan for the recording session as much as possible beforehand.
- Anticipate potential problems and possible appropriate solutions.
- Allow plenty of time to set up.
- Know the audio system well to get the best from it.
- Test all aspects of the system prior to the start of the session.
- Approach problems in a methodical and logical manner and consider possible alternative solutions before deciding on a course of action.
- Experiment to the get best results out of a particular setup or scenario.

- Respect the performers/artists, communicate effectively with them, and consider their own opinions in order to achieve the best possible results.

And finally, at all times listen carefully to the audio material: develop your listening skills, learn to trust your ears, and make an honest evaluation as to the quality of the final results in a bid to make even better vocal recordings in the future.

FURTHER READING

Bartlett. B., & Bartlett, J. (2005). *Practical recording techniques: The step-by-step approach to professional studio recording* (4th ed.). Oxford, UK: Focal Press.

Eargle, J. (2004). *The microphone book: From mono to stereo to surround—A guide to microphone design and application* (2nd ed.). Oxford, UK: Focal Press.

Granqvist, S., & Svec, J. G. (2005, September*). Microphones and room acoustics and their influence on voice signals.* Paper presented at PEVoC 6, London Retrieved from http://www.speech.kth.se/~svante/Granqvist_Svec_PEVoC6_Microphones.ppt

Howard, D. M., & Angus, J. A. S. (2006). *Acoustics and psychoacoustics* (3rd ed.). Oxford, UK: Focal Press.

Hugonnet, C., & Walder, P. (1998). *Stereophonic sound recording, Theory and practice.* Chichester, UK: John Wiley and Sons.

Jers, H., & Ternström, S. (2004, June). *Intonation analysis of a multi-channel choir recording.* Paper presented at the Baltic-Nordic Acoustics Meeting, Mariehamn, Åland, Finland.

Rumsey, F., & McCormick, T. (2005). *Sound and recording—An introduction* (5th ed.). Oxford, UK: Focal Press.

Talbot-Smith, M. (2004). *Sound engineering explained* (2nd ed.). Oxford, UK: Focal Press.

Talbot-Smith, M. (2004). *Sound engineer's pocket book* (2nd ed.). Oxford, UK: Focal Press.

APPENDIX 1

Glossary

Acceptance angle: Useful region of frontal pickup for a directional microphone or stereo pair, defined as an angular range ± 0 degrees for which the level of an on-axis sound source is between ± 3dB. Beyond this angular range the microphone will be less than ideal in terms of its frequency response due to off-axis colorization.

ADT (automatic double tracking): Simulates the effect of recording a musician playing the same part twice on two separate tracks. It uses a short delay to simulate the timing variations.

Affricate: A speech sound that combines a plosive with a fricative, such as the consonants in *each* and *jaw*.

Alto: Short for contralto—the lowest of the female singing voices.

Amplifier: An electronic circuit that increases the level of a signal.

Analog: In this case refers to a signal (e.g., electrical, magnetic) that directly represents an acoustic signal. Analog media (such as vinyl or cassettes) make a permanent record of the sound using a continuously varying signal.

Anechoic: A reflection-free and therefore reverberation-free room or environment.

Articulation: Moving those parts of the vocal tract (e.g., tongue, lips, and jaw) that change its shape and volume.

Atto-: Prefix indicating a million million millionth, or 10^{-18}.

Balanced: An audio connection which uses two signal wires and a screen that carries no signal. Any interference is picked up equally by the two wires and effectively canceled at the balanced input connection stage. Capable of carrying phantom power and useful for long cable runs with minimal signal loss.

Baritone: The male singing range between the bass and tenor.

Bass: The lowest male singing voice.

Bel: A tenth of a decibel.

Castrato: A male singer with a soprano singing range due to castration prior to pubertal voice transformation.

CD (compact disc): A popular digital recording format, first appearing in 1982, surpassing vinyl record sales in 1988. Two-track, using a sample rate of 44.1 kHz and a resolution of 16 bits.

CD-R (CD-recordable): A digital data storage format, based on the same technology as the audio CD. It is used to store and distribute up to 700 MB of data files or audio material.

Centi-: Prefix indicating a hundredth, or 10^{-2}.

Channel: A strip of vertical controls in a mixing desk relating to a single mono audio signal input or sometimes a double stereo input.

Clipping: The unpleasant effect that is achieved when a signal exceeds the dynamic range of the medium being used. In analog systems this is sometimes desirable in terms of the perceptual effect it has on the audio material. With a digital system clipping occurs when the signal exceeds 0 dB FS and results in very harsh distortion. Also known as *distortion* or *clipping distortion*.

Closed phase: The portion of the vocal fold vibration cycle for which the folds are in contact, often referred to as *CP*.

Closed quotient: The percentage of a vocal fold vibration cycle for which the folds are in contact, often referred to as *CQ*.

Coincident pair: A stereo microphone technique where two separate microphones are placed so that their diaphragms occupy approximately the same point in space. They are angled apart and placed so that one is directly on top of the other. Also known as a *crossed pair*, *XY*, or *normal stereo*. The technique is based on the level time.

Complex nonperiodic waveform: A waveform that exhibits no repeating pattern or cycle.

Complex periodic waveform: A nonsinusoidal waveform that exhibits a repeating pattern or cycle.

Compressor: A device designed to alter the dynamic characteristics of an audio signal by reducing signal peaks so that the overall level can be boosted without clipping. Hence, it acts to make the loudest parts of the signal quieter and the quieter aspects louder.

Condenser microphone: A microphone that works on the principle of variable capacitance to generate an electrical signal.

Contralto: See *alto*.

Countertenor: A male singing voice in the alto range that is primarily based on falsetto.

Creaky voice: A voice quality that is low and rather broken up in pitch, in which the vocal folds are relaxed and vibrating at a low frequency, often with more than one closure per cycle.

Crescendo: A gradual increase in loudness.

Critical distance: The sound source to listener distance at which the levels of the direct sound and the reverberant field are equal. Also known as the reverberation radius.

Cycle: The pattern that is repeated in a periodic waveform.

DAT (digital audio tape): A tape-based digital recording medium, introduced in 1987, but mostly used in studios. Two-track, 16 bit, and usually 48 kHz.

dB: See *decibel*.

dB (SIL): Decibel level based on a sound intensity level measurement.

dB (SPL): Decibel level based on a sound pressure level measurement.

Deci-: Prefix indicating a tenth, or 10^{-1}.

Decibel: A dimensionless unit used for measuring sound intensity or sound pressure level. The decibel measurement is a ratio measurement that indicates how loud a sound level is with respect to a reference (usually the softest sound that can, on average, be heard). Shorthand is *dB*.

Decrescendo: A gradual decrease in loudness.

De-esser: A frequency selective compressor designed to minimize vocal sibilance.

Diaphragm: A large muscle beneath the lungs that is the main one used for breathing.

Digital: Refers to a signal which is coded as a stream of binary numbers. When sound is digitized, the original analog signal is sampled many times per second and each sample is represented as a binary number. The result can therefore be easily stored and manipulated as part of a computer system.

Directivity pattern: The directional characteristics of a microphone, shown as a polar plot with angle of incidence vs. amplitude. An omnidirectional microphone favors no particular angle and so has a theoretically perfectly circular directivity pattern. Also known as a *polar pickup patter* or just *polar plot*.

Ducker: A type of compressor where another trigger signal is used to control the signal level of the compressor input. Used in public address systems to attenuate backing music, etc., during an announcement.

DVD (digital versatile disc): A high-density recording medium, introduced in 1996 and used for films and computer data storage. Derivatives also include DVD-audio and the latest, HD-DVD (high-definition DVD).

Dynamic microphone: A microphone that generates an electrical signal when acoustic pressure waves cause a conductive coil to vibrate in a stationary magnetic field.

Dynamic range: The difference in dB SPL between the maximum acceptable level and noise floor of a system or microphone, being the useful variation between the quietest and loudest acoustic signals that a microphone or system can reasonably deal with.

Dynamics: Refers to the softness or loudness of an audio signal and its related variation over time. A dynamic audio signal is said to show significant variation between the loudest and softest parts, and this is very evident when viewed as a waveform.

Electret: A type of condenser microphone in which the electrostatic charge on the plates of the capacitor is generated by an electret—a material that permanently stores an electrostatic charge.

Electroglottograph: See *electrolaryngography*.

Electroglottography: See *electrolaryngography*.

Electrolaryngograph: See *electrolaryngography*.

Electrolaryngography: A technique that allows vocal fold contact area to be monitored against time by measuring the current flowing between two electrodes that are placed externally on the neck at the level of the larynx (electrolaryngography uses an electrolaryngograph, and electroglottography uses an electroglottograph). The key difference between electrolaryngography and electroglottography is that the output waveform of the former is plotted with vocal fold closure going vertically, while that for the latter is plotted with vocal fold closure going negatively.

ENT: Ear, nose, and throat.

Equalization: Frequency selective gain, defined by center frequency control, cut or boost applied, Q factor, and bandwidth. Typical examples are shelving, parametric, graphic, etc.

Exa-: Prefix indicating a million million million, or 10^{18}.

f0: Shorthand for fundamental frequency.

Falsetto: A voice quality that has a high fundamental frequency that is achieved by restricting the vibrating portions of the vocal folds.

Feedback: Acoustic feedback occurs when, for instance, a microphone signal is amplified and played back from a loudspeaker, picked up by the microphone again, and played back through the amplifier and speaker system again. The loop continues and results in a high pitched and unpleasant squeal if left unchecked, corresponding to a particular resonant frequency characteristic of the audio system in question.

Femto-: Prefix indicating a thousand million millionth, or 10^{-15}.

Foldback: An audio signal usually differing from what the audience or sound engineer will hear, which is specifically created and presented to a performer during recording or when using a PA system so that he can hear himself over other nearby sound sources.

Formant: An acoustic resonance of the vocal tract; usually, four to eight formants are considered in acoustic analysis of speech or singing, which are labeled first formant (F1), second formant (F2), etc., and their center frequencies, or *formant frequencies*, change as the vocal tract shape is altered.

Formant frequency: The center frequency of a formant.

Formant tuning: An enhancement in the energy of a sung output achieved by moving a formant so that it lies over or very close to the frequency of a harmonic.

Frequency response: How the gain in a system varies with frequency.

Fricative: A speech sound, such as the consonants in *Sue, zoo, show, Joe, fee,* and *vee,* that involves acoustic noise as its voice source (voiceless fricatives) and acoustic noise as well as vocal fold vibration (voiced fricatives), resulting from the airstream flowing through a narrow gap in the vocal tract.

Front of house (FOH): That aspect of a PA system that relates to the audience. The FOH mixing desk is located in the audience so that the engineer can hear what the audience hears. The FOH speakers are those used to project sound to the audience rather than the performers.

Fundamental frequency: The number of repeating cycles of a periodic waveform occurring in one second. The unit is the Hertz or Hz and the common shorthand is *f0*.

Gate: A device that attenuates or stops a signal from being heard unless it is above a specific level threshold. Also known as a noise gate.

Giga-: Prefix indicating a thousand million, or 10^9.

Glottal stop: The sudden release of a glottal closure.

Glottis: The space between the vocal folds.

Harmonic: A spectral component of a complex periodic waveform. Each harmonic is an integer (1, 2, 3, 4 . . .) multiple of the fundamental frequency.

ILD: Interaural level difference. Spatial hearing mechanism based on level differences between our ears. Works for higher frequency sounds only. Leads to the development of coincident microphone techniques.

Intensity: Power per unit area.

ITD: Interaural time difference. Spatial hearing mechanism based on time differences between our ears. Works for lower frequency sounds only.

Leads to the development of spaced microphone techniques.

Kilo-: Prefix indicating a thousand, or 10^3.

Larynx: The organ in the neck that is used for voiced sounds; sometimes referred to as the *voice box*.

Limiter: A specific type of compressor designed to stop a signal from crossing a particular threshold to avoid clipping distortion.

Line level: Signals at a nominal level of −10 dBV to +4 dBu, generally from a powered electrical audio device such as a synthesizer, CD player, or effects unit.

Long-term average spectrum: An average of a number of short-term spectra.

Loudness: The perceived level of a sound which changes as acoustic intensity changes.

LTAS: Long-term average spectrum.

Manner: A description used (with voice and place) to describe the way in which speech sounds are articulated.

Microphone: A device that converts sound pressure variations into an electrical voltage signal.

Mega-: Prefix indicating a million, or 10^6.

Mezzo-soprano: The female singing voice that is between an alto and a soprano.

Micro-: Prefix indicating a millionth, or 10^{-6}.

Milli-: Prefix indicating a thousandth, or 10^{-3}.

Monitor: Generally refers to listening to the output of an audio system. Hence, loudspeakers are sometimes called monitors. Also that aspect of a PA system that relates to the on-stage performers. The monitor mixing desk in a large PA system is located on or near the stage. The monitor speakers (also known as wedges) are those used to project sound to the performers rather than the audience.

Multicore: A cable with multiple individual cores, allowing many audio signals to be carried independently but as part of one.

Nano-: Prefix indicating a thousand millionth, or 10^{-9}.

Nasal cavity: Nose.

Noise gate: A device that attenuates or stops a signal from being heard unless it is above a specific level threshold. Also known as a *gate*.

Nonvoiced sounds: See *voiceless sounds*.

Omnidirectional: A microphone directivity pattern that is perfectly uniform; that is, the microphone is equally responsive to sounds incident from any angle.

Open phase: The portion of the vocal fold vibration cycle for which the folds are apart, often referred to as *OP*.

Open quotient: The percentage of a vocal fold vibration cycle for which the folds are apart, often referred to as *OQ*.

Oral cavity: Mouth.

Overtones: Harmonics that are *over* the fundamental, where the first overtone is the first tone over the fundamental (the second harmonic), the second overtone is the third harmonic, etc.

Period: The time that a repeating cycle lasts.

Peta-: Prefix indicating a thousand million million, or 10^{15}.

Phantom power: 12 to 48 v DC applied to pins 2 and 3 of the microphone connector required to make non-electret condenser microphones work. Usually supplied from the microphone input of the mixing desk, but can also come from an internal battery. Although only used for condenser type microphones, phantom power will not damage the internal workings of a dynamic microphone if used in error.

Pharynx: The vocal tract region between the larynx and the velum.

Phase cancellation: Occurs when two acoustic (or electric) signals are added together that are not exactly matched —hence, are not in phase. Peaks and troughs in the signal waveform do not line up, and this can result in a signal of lower amplitude than the original, or additional peaks or troughs in the overall frequency response. Typically occurs when a signal plus a very slightly delayed version of the same signal are added together. Hence, may happen due to reflections from a surface being added to the direct sound at a microphone or due to timing differences when using multiple spaced microphones.

Phonation: A sound with a sound source that involves vocal fold vibration.

Phono: A one signal wire plus screen hi-fi connector carrying a line level signal and used extensively on semiprofessional recording equipment.

Pico-: Prefix indicating a million millionth, or 10^{-12}.

Pitch: The perception of tones on a scale from low to high, essentially, but not entirely, due to changes in fundamental frequency.

Place: A description used (with voice and manner) to describe where in the vocal tract speech sounds are articulated.

Plosive: A speech sound that involves a complete vocal tract closure behind which lung air pressure builds up, and the closure is released to create the characteristic sound.

Polar pickup pattern: See *directivity pattern*.

Power source: In the context of voice production, the energy source for sound creation, which is provided from the lungs as an outflow of air by the breathing mechanism.

Preamp: An electronic circuit and the first stage of amplification used to boost a signal level. Found in the input stages of mixing desk for boosting microphone levels, also as external stand-alone units and as part of the internal workings of a condenser microphone.

Proximity effect: The bass boost that occurs when using a cardioid type microphone placed close to a sound source. The closer the microphone, the greater the low frequency boost.

Public address (PA) system: An audio system consisting of microphone(s), a mixing desk, and usually audio effects processors, together with amplification and loudspeakers for presenting audio material to a wider audience or across a large venue. Will also include amplification and loudspeakers to provide foldback for on-stage performers.

Resonance: A preferred frequency of a system, which in the case of the vocal tract is the set of formants associated with different articulations that create various vocal tract shapes during speech and singing.

Reverberation radius: The sound source to listener distance at which the levels of the direct sound and the reverberant field are equal. Also known as the *critical distance*.

Sensitivity: The unloaded output voltage of a microphone determined by placing it in front of a reference sound source with a measured sound pressure level of 94 dB at 1 kHz. This value for SPL is the same as a pressure value of 1 Pa.

Short-term spectrum: A single spectrum.

Signal to noise ratio: The ratio between the measured noise floor or noise level of a medium and a reference signal transmitted through this medium; typically for microphones, a 1 kHz test tone at 94 dB SPL.

SIL: Sound intensity level.

Singer's formant: A resonance in the 2.5 kHz to 4 kHz region that gives a voice projection over an orchestra, often described as its *ring*.

Soprano: The female singing voice above a mezzo-soprano.

Sound modifiers: The cavities of the vocal tract which lie between the sound source and the lips and/or nostrils.

Sound source: The mechanism that converts power from the power source into sound, which in speech is either the vibrating vocal folds for voiced sounds, or air being forced past a constriction in the vocal tract for a voiceless sound.

Spectrum: A plot of energy against frequency. A single spectrum is known as a *short-term* spectrum, and an average of a number of short-term spectra is known as a *long-term average spectrum*, or *LTAS*.

Spectrogram: The output plot from a spectrograph, which is plotted either in color or greyscale with frequency on the vertical axis, time on the horizontal axis, and the color or degree of grey indicating the energy level at that frequency at that point in time.

Spectrograph: A machine or computer program that carries out an analysis of the energy in an acoustic signal across frequency and time. The output, known as a *spectrogram*, is plotted either in color or greyscale with frequency on the vertical axis, time on the horizontal axis, and the color or degree of grey indicating the energy level at that frequency at that point in time.

SPL: Sound pressure level.

Stereo image: A sound image generated by amplitude panning so that it emanates from between two stereo speakers rather than directly from a single speaker.

Support: A term employed by voice teachers to indicate control of the power source from the region of the diaphragm.

Tenor: The male singing voice above the baritone and below the countertenor.

Tera-: Prefix indicating a million million, or 10^{12}.

Timbre: A perceived difference between sounds that is not related to a change in pitch, loudness, or duration.

Transient: A short-lived signal, or part of a signal.

Two-track: An audio recording that uses two separate tracks of sound—usually to produce stereo. Typical media include CD, cassette, vinyl, DAT, minidisk.

Unbalanced: An audio connection which uses one signal wire and a screen, which carries no signal. Cannot carry phantom power and is susceptible to noise over long cable runs.

VCA (voltage controlled amplifier): An electronic amplifier that varies its gain depending on a control voltage. Used in an audio compressor.

Velum: The soft palate, which can be moved up to close off the nasal cavity from the airstream and down to open it.

Vibrato: Periodic modulation of the fundamental frequency often associated with operatic singing.

Vocal chords: A popular (but misunderstood) term for the vocal cords or vocal folds.

Vocal cords: Another term for vocal folds.

Vocal folds: The vibrating muscles in the larynx that provide the sound source during voiced sounds.

Vocal tract: The oral cavity (mouth) and nasal cavity (nose).

Voice: 1. A description used (with place and manner) to describe whether a speech sound is voiced or voiceless. 2. The sound made by the human vocal instrument.

Voice box: Common popular term for the larynx.

Voiced sounds: Sounds in speech or singing that involve the vibrating vocal folds.

Voiceless sounds: Sounds in speech or singing that do not involve the vibrating vocal folds, sometimes referred to as *nonvoiced sounds*.

Waveform: A plot of a measured quantity against time.

Wavelength: The length of one cycle of a periodic disturbance in space, usually given the Greek letter lambda (λ).

Whistle register: The highest female singing voice which can extend to over two and a half octaves above middle C.

XLR: 3-pin male/female balanced audio connector used (among other things) to connect microphones to mixer inputs. Capable of carrying phantom power.

Yocto-: Prefix indicating a million million million millionth, or 10^{-24}.

Yotta-: Prefix indicating a million million million million, or 10^{24}.

Zepto-: Prefix indicating a thousand million million millionth, or 10^{-21}.

Zetta-: Prefix indicating a thousand million million million, or 10^{21}.

APPENDIX 2

Power Source (Breathing) Flip Book

(© Voice Matters Ltd, http://www.voicematters.org.uk; used with permission.)

To make the power source (breathing) flip book:

1. Photocopy three copies of the following page so that your original book is not damaged.
    Choose heavier than normal paper if available to prolong the life of the flip book.
2. Cut along the dotted lines with scissors.
    Do be very careful when using scissors; ask for help as appropriate.
3. Stack the pages in order (here this is 123412341234).
4. Put a staple through the stack where the word staple is printed or use glue.
    Do be careful with a stapling machine or glue and follow manufacturer's instructions.

To use the book, grip around the staple between the thumb and forefinger of one hand, and flip the pages with the thumb of the other hand. You will see an animated breathing sequence.

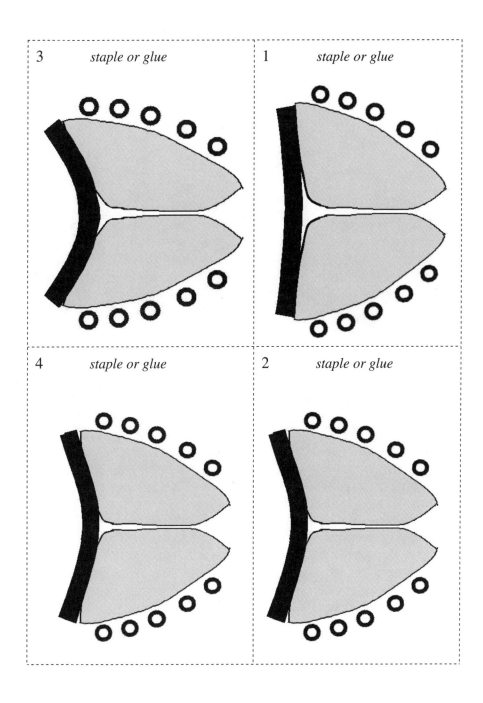

3   *staple or glue*

1   *staple or glue*

4   *staple or glue*

2   *staple or glue*

APPENDIX 3

Sound Source
(Vocal Fold Vibration)
Flip Book

(© Voice Matters Ltd, http://www.voicematters.org.uk; used with permission.)

To make the sound source (vocal fold vibration) flip book, follow instructions for construction given in Appendix 2.

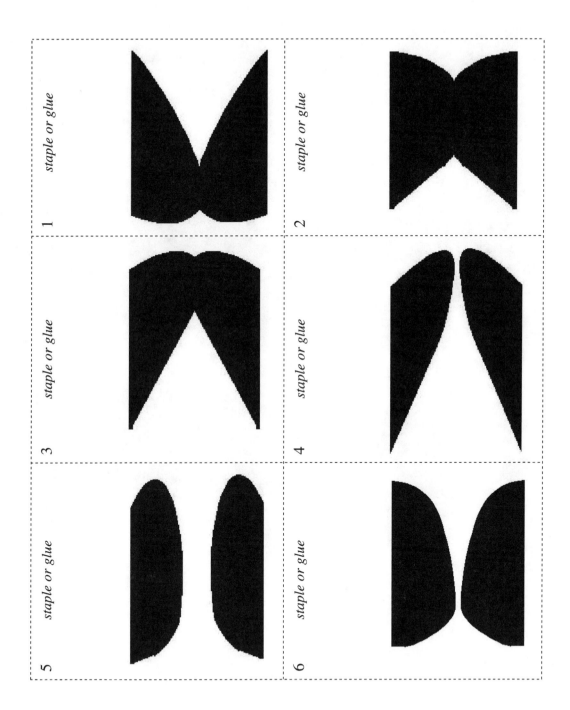

APPENDIX 4

Sound Modifier (Oral Tract Area) Flip Book

To make the sound modifier (oral tract area) flip book, which is for the diphthong in I (SAMPA: /aI/), follow instructions for construction given in Appendix 2.

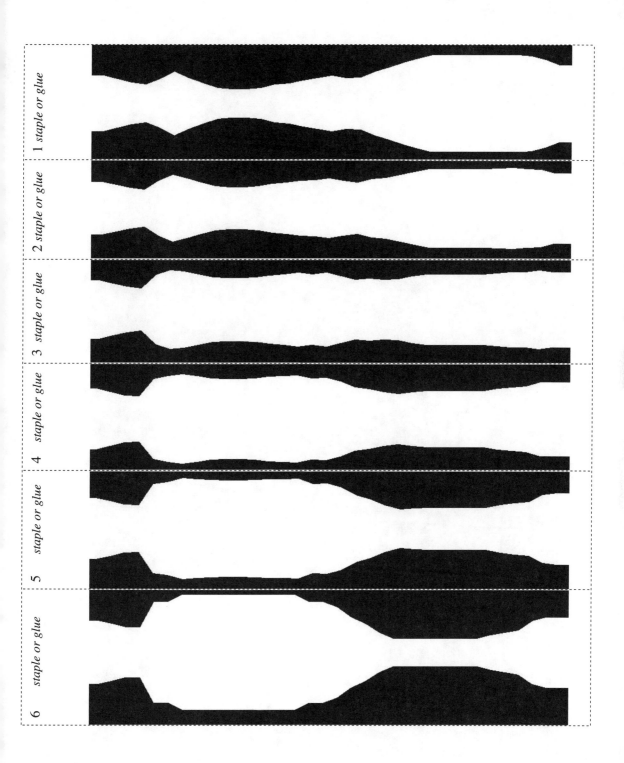

staple or glue   1

staple or glue   2

staple or glue   3

staple or glue   4

staple or glue   5

staple or glue   6

Index

Note: Page numbers in **bold** reference non-text material.

A

Absorption values, acoustics, **79**
Acceptance angle, 100
Acoustic advantage
    performing to best in a space, 85–91
    working space for best, 86–88
Acoustic labyrinth, 100
Acoustic output, 38–56
    power/sound source, 38–44
        mixed, 40
        voiced, 39–40
        voiceless, 40
Acoustic pressure, 5–6
    waveforms, 9, 10
Acoustic screens, 89–90
Acoustic signature, 76
Acoustic wave transmission, effect of
        environment on, 68
Acoustical resistance, 100
Acoustically porous, 79
    effects, **83**
Acoustics
    absorption values, **79**
    effect of room on, **69**
    of spaces, 68–78
        modifying, 78–85
    of surface materials, 78–80
Adam's apple, 30
Adduction, vocal folds, 30
ADR (Automatic dialogue replacement),
        162
ADT (Automatic double tracking), 155
Affricates
    defined, 38
    sound modifiers, 50

Alexander technique, 60
Amplitude, defined, 10, 74
Anechoic
    chamber, **163**
    recording, 162–164
    room, 68
Anti-resonance, defined, 49
Aperiodic waveforms, 10
Articulation
    phoneme, 34
        manner, 38
        place, 34–36
Artificial reverberation, 128–129
    parameters, 129–130
    setting up, 129–130
Aspiration, 48
Audio compression, setting up, 123–127
Audio compressor, 122–123
Audio signal, path of, **94**
Automatic dialogue replacement (ADR),
        162
Automatic double tracking (ADT), 155
Aux send effects, dynamics processor,
        127–130
Auxiliary masters, 121
Auxiliary section, voice recording
        systems and, 117–119
Average spectra, 12–15

B

Background vocals, recording, 176–177
Bass, defined, 72
Bel scale, 18
Bell, Alexander Graham, decibels and, 18

Bernoulli effect, defined, 30–32
Blumlein, Alan, 166
Blumlein pair, 165–166
Bone conduction, defined, 72
Boundary microphone, 171
Breathing, physics of, 26–27
Burst, center frequency, 47
Byte, defined, 3

C

Cardioid directivity pattern, 99–100
Cardioid microphones, 107
    vs. omnidirectional microphones,
        multiple soloists and, 172
Coincident stereo
    described, 165
    microphone recording, 165–168
Communications
    environment impact on, 67–68
    during recording sessions, 151
Complete acoustic waveforms, 9
Complex periodic waveforms, 10, 13
Computers, in voice training, 56–59
Condenser microphones vs. dynamic
        microphones, 95–98
Consonant sounds, **35**, 47
CQ (closed quotient)
    larynx, 43–44
    training enhancements, 44
Creaky voice qualities, 43
Critical distance, 77
Cycle, defined, 10

D

De-essing, 153
    described, 154–155
Decibels (dB), 18–21
    sound pressure levels in, **20**
Diaphragm, function of, 28–29
Digital audio workstation, 133
Diphthongs, **37**
    acoustics of, 47
Direct sound
    levels of, **77**
    relative sound of, 76
Directivity index, 101

Directivity patterns, microphones, 98–102
Distance factor, 101
Drinks, healthy voice and, 61–62
Ducking, defined, 159–160
Dynamic microphones, 95–97, 97
    vs. condenser microphones, 95–98
Dynamic range, 106
Dynamics processor
    aux send effects, 127–130
    gating, 127
    setting up, 123–127

E

Early reflections, reverb, 130
Early sound, defined, 73–75
Effects returns, 121–122
Electret microphones, 96
Electromagnetic induction, 95
Ensemble recording, 173–176
    microphone selection/placement of,
        174–175
    potential problems, 175
Environment
    effect on acoustic pressure wave
        transmission, 68
    impact on communications, 67–68
    sound modification effect on, 68
Equalization (EQ) controls
    fixed or shelving, 115
    graphic, 115–116
    microphone preamp stage, 114–117
    notch filter, 116–117
    paragraphic, 116
    parametric, 115
    semiparametric, 115
Exabytes (Eb), defined, 5
Exponential decay, 74

F

Fader
    master, 121
    voice recording systems and, 119–120
Farads, 5
Feedback
    elimination of, 141
    loop, 141

Feldenkrais technique, 60
Figure-of-eight directivity pattern, microphones, 99, 107–108
Float microphone, 171
Flutter echoes, 87
Foldback, 43, 89–90, 117–118
  mix, for studio recording, 151
  reflectors and, 90
Food, healthy voice and, 61–62
Format transitions
  defined, 48
  idealized plots, **48**
Fourier components, defined, 10
Fourier theorem, mathematics, 13
Frequency (f), defined, 8
Frequency components, defined, 10
Frequency dependent compressor diagram, **154**
Frequency response, microphones, 102–105
Fricatives
  defined, 30, 38
  sound modifiers, 49–50
Front-of-house (FOH) mixing desk, 134
Fundamental frequency (f0), 10

G

Gated reverb, 130
Gigabyte (Gb), defined, 3
Glottis, defined, 30
Graphic EQ, 115–116
Group outputs, voice recording systems and, 120–127

H

Harmonic number, 11
Harmonics, 10–12
  defined, 17
Head movement, stereo recording and, 165
Head, shadow effect of human, 70
Hertz (Hz), defined, 8
High-pass/low-cut filter, microphone preamp stage, 112–113
Hypercardioid directivity pattern, 100–102

I

ILD (Interaural level difference), 165
Input connection, 111
Input pulse, displacement, 5
Insert effects, 122
Insert point, mixing desk and, 113–114
Inspiratory intercostals, 28
Interaural level difference (ILD), 165
Interaural time difference (ITD), 164
Internal labyrinth, 100
ITD (Interaural time difference), 164

K

Kilobyte (kb), defined, 3

L

Larynx
  tilting mechanism, **31**
  voice production and, 29
Larynx closed quotient (CQ), 43–44
Line microphones, 101
Line spectrum, defined, 13
Live recording
  effects processing, 158
  on location, 160–162
    microphone selection/placement of, 160–161
  microphone selection/placement of, 156–157
    on location, 160–162
  potential problems, 157–158
  spoken word, 158–160
    effects processing, 162
    potential problems, 161–162
  voice reinforcement, 155–158
Location
  recording on, 160–162
    microphone selection/placement of, 160–161
Locus, 48
Long-term average spectra (LTAS), 14–15
  spectrograms, **59**
Long-term spectra, 12–15
Longitudinal wave, 6
Looping, 162

M

Master fader, 121
Master section, voice recording systems and, 120–127
Megabyte (Mb), defined, 3
Metering, 127
Mic/line input, microphones, 110–111
Microfarad (µf), defined, 5
Microphone preamp stage, voice recording systems, 108–113
Microphones, 94–108
  boundary, 171
  cardioid, 107
    directivity pattern and, 99–100
  directivity patterns, 98–102
  dynamic vs. condenser, 95–98
  ensemble recording and, 174–175
  figure-of-eight directivity pattern, 99, 107–108
  frequency response, 102–105
  hypercardioid directivity pattern and, 100–102
  input connection, 111
  maximum acceptable level, 106
  mic/line input, 110–111
  microphone selection/placement for, 151–153
  noise, 106
  omnidirectional, 98–99, 107
  overload point, 106
  preamp stage, 108–113
  pressure, 99
  recording for research and, 149–150
  selection/placement of, 150
    for live recording, 156–157
  sensitivity, 105–106
  spaced techniques, 168–169
  supercardioid, 101
    directivity pattern and, 100–102
  use of, 107
Mid-side (M-S) recording, 167
Millifarad (mf), defined, 5
Milliseconds (ms), 7
Mixed sound source, 30, 39
Mixing desk
  channel, **109**
  front-of-house, 134
  insert point and, 113–114

Modal voice qualities, Modal, 43
Monophthongs, **37**
  acoustics of, 45
  defined, 47
Moving-coil microphones. *See* Dynamic microphones
Multiple soloists. *See* Soloists, multiple
  ensemble recording, 173–176
  omnidirectional vs. cardioid microphones, 172
  source/location of, 173–174
  source separation/background noise, 172
Multiplying factors, **4**
Myoelastic aerodynamic theory of vocal fold vibration, 32

N

Narrow-band spectrogram, 16
Nasal cavity, 33
Nasal murmur, 49
Nasal sound modifiers, 49
Noise
  extraneous on stage, 157
  microphones, 106
Nonperiodic waveforms, 10
Notch filter, equalization (EQ) and, 116–117
Numbers
  equivalent powers of ten, **4**
  multiplying factors, **4**
  prefixes, **4**
  scientific use of, 3–5
  symbols for, **4**

O

Omnidirectional microphones, 98–99, 107
  vs. cardioid microphones, multiple soloists and, 172
Oral cavity, defined, 33
Outdoor recording. *See* Recording, on location
Overload point, microphones, 106

P

Pad, microphone preamp stage, 112
Pan (Panoramic potentiometer), voice recording systems and, 119

Paragraphic EQ, 116
Parametric EQ, 115
Performance, considerations for vocal, 88–91
Performance space, visual considerations, 86
Period (T), 7
  defined, 10
Perturbation theory, 51–53
Petabytes (Pb), defined, 5
Phantom power, 97, 111
Phase, 11
  cancellation, defined, 151
  microphone preamp stage, 113
Phoneme articulation, 34
  manner, 38
  place, 36–38
Piano, f0 ranges in, **41**
Picofarad (pf), defined, 5
Pinnae cues, 165
Pitch, defined, 10
Plate reverb, 129
Plosives, 47–49
  defined, 38
Point masses, 5
Polar plot, 98
Pop shields, making/positioning, 153
Post processing, 76
Post-synchro, 162
Powers of ten, **4**
Pre-delay, reverb, 129
Presence peak, 104
Preset, reverb, 129
Pressure microphone, 99
Prevoicing, defined, 34, 49
Proximity effect, 104
Public address system, **135**
  defined, 134
  for large venues, **139**
  for medium venues, **137**
Pure tone, 10

R

Reach, defined, 101
Recording
  background vocals, 176–177
  communications during, 151
  ensemble, 173–174, 175–176

    microphone selection/placement of, 175–176
    potential problems, 175–176
  live
    effects processing, 158
    on location, 160–162, 162
    microphone selection/placement of, 156–157, 160–161
    potential problems, 157–158
    reinforcement of vocal, 155–158
  multiple sources
    coincident stereo microphone recording, 165–168
    head movement and, 165
    interaural level difference (ILD), 165
    interaural time difference (ITD), 164
    pinnae cues, 165
  use of reverberation, 76
  vocal, multiple soloists, 169–173
  voice
    anechoic, 162–164
    microphone selection/placement of, 149–153
    from multiple sources, 164–177
  see also Voice recording
Recording for research, 149–155
  microphone selection for, 149–150
Recording systems
  medium, 130–133
    analog, 130–131
    digital, 131–132
    linear, 132
    multitrack, 132
    nonlinear, 132
    two-track (stereo), 132
  voice, 108–133
    auxiliary section, 117–119
    microphone preamp stage, 108–113
Reflectors, Foldback and, 90
Relative sound, of direct sound, 76
Research
  recording for, 149–155
    microphone selection for, 149–150
Reverb, 128–129
  parameters, 129–130
  setting up, 129–130
  time, 130
Reverberant field, 74
  buildup of, **75**

Reverberant sound, defined, 73–76
Reverberation time (RT$_{60}$), 74
  calculating, for a room, 80–84
Reverse reverb, 129
Ribbon microphones, 96–98
Rifle microphones, 101
Room
  calculating reverberation time for, 80–84
  effect of on acoustics, **69**
Routing, voice recording systems and, 119

S

Sabin values, 80
SAMPA (Speech Assessment
    Methodologies Phonetic
    Alphabet), symbols, **35**
Self-monitoring, 88–89
Semiparametric EQ, 115
Semivowels
  defined, 38
  sound modifiers, 50–51
Sensitivity, microphones, 105–106
Shadow effect, of human head, 70
Short-term spectra, 12–15
Shotgun microphones, 101
Signal-to-noise ratio, defined, 106
Sine waveforms, 10–12
  plot of, **11**
Singer's formant, 55
Singing
  f0 ranges in, **41**
  formants in, 53–56
Single vocal sources
  voice recording, 149–164
    for research, 149–155
Soft palate, 34
Soloists, multiple
  ensemble recording, 173–176
  off-axis colorization, 172
  omnidirectional vs. cardioid
    microphones, 172
  phase cancellation effects, 172–173
  recording, 169–173
  source/location of, 173–174
  source separation/background noise, 5,
    172
Sound
  buildup, 74

  check, 144–145
  decay, 74
  energy half life, 74
  fricatives modifiers, 49–50
  input, 68
  level maintenance, 144-145
  output, 68
  source, into a space, 69–72
  in steady state, 74
Sound modifiers, 68
  affricates, 50
  defined, 45
  modified by space, 72–74
  output from space, 75–78
  nasals, 49
  plosives, 47–49
  pressure levels, in decibels, **20**
  recording, audiopath of, **94**
  reinforcement of vocal, 133–145
    large venues, 138
    medium sized venues, 137–138
    operational guidelines, 138–145
    small venues, 134–136
  semivowels, 50–51
  source of, 5, 68
  speed of, 7
  transmission of, 5
    point mass/spring model of, **6**
    two dimensional, **7**
  unwanted, 69, **70**
  in voice production, 33–34
  velocity of, 7
  vowels, 45–47
  wanted, 69, **70**
  wave, 6
Sound reinforcement
  defined, 133
  live, 155–158
    microphone placement, 156–157
  vocal, 133–145
    large venues, 138
    medium sized venues, 137–138
    operational guidelines, 138–145
    small venues, 134–136
Space, sound output from, 75–78
Spaced microphone techniques, 168–169
Spaces
  acoustics of, 68–78
  modifying, 78–85

changing surface materials in, 84–85
performing to best acoustic advantage
        in, 85–91
sound modification by, 72–74
sound source into, 69–72
visual considerations, 86
Spectra, average, 12–15
Spectrograms, 15–18
    defined, 16
    long-term average spectra (LTAS), **59**
    narrowband, **59**
Spectrum, defined, 13
Speech Assessment Methodologies
        Phonetic Alphabet (SAMPA)
    described, 34
    symbols, **35**
Speech, f0 ranges in, **41**
Speech intelligibility, 77
Speed, of sound, 7
Spoken word
    live recording, 158–160
        effects processing, 162
        potential problems, 161–162
Stereo recording
    multiple sources
        coincident stereo microphone
            recording, 165–168
        head movement and, 165
        interaural level difference (ILD), 165
        interaural time difference (ITD), 164
        pinnae cues, 165
    spaced microphone techniques,
        168–169
Stops, defined, 38
Striations, defined, 17
Studio voice recording, 150–151
    effects processing, 153–155
    live sound reinforcement, 155–158
    problems, 153
Supercardioid directivity pattern, 100–102
Supercardioid microphones, 101
Surface materials, acoustics of, 78–80
Swept mid EQ, 115

T

Talkback, 122
Terabytes (Tb), defined, 3
Timbre, defined, 10

Transverse wave, 6
Traveling wave, 6
Treble, defined, 72
Trim/gain, recording systems and,
        111–112

U

Unwanted sound, defined, 69, **70**

V

Velocity, 5–8
    of sound, 7
Velum, 34
Verbal performance, room acoustics and,
        69
Vibration, vocal folds, 30–33
Visual considerations, spaces, 86
Vocal folds
    adduction, 30
    myoelastic aerodynamic theory of
        vibration of, 32
    vibration, 30–33
    voice production and, 29
Vocal output
    acoustics of, 38–56
        power/sound source, 38–44
Vocal performance considerations, 88–91
Vocal sound reinforcement, 133–145
    operational guidelines, 138–145
    venues
        large, 138
        medium sized, 137–138
        small, 134–136
Voice, 34, 36
    developing and maintaining healthy,
        56–64
    healthy
        environmental considerations, 62–63
        food and drink and, 61–62
    training using computers, 56–59
    warm-up/cool-down, 60–61
Voice box, voice production and, 29
Voice onset time (VOT), defined, 48
Voice production
    larynx and, 29
    power source, power source, 26–29
    sound modifiers in, 33–34

Voice production *(continued)*
  sound source in, 29–33
  vocal folds and, 29
  voice box and, 29
Voice qualities, 42
  creaky, 43
  falsetto, 43
  modal voice, 43
Voice recording
  anechoic, 162–164
  application of, 148–149
  environment for, 148
  listener and, 148–149
  microphone selection for, 149–150
  multiple soloists, 169–173
  multiple sources, 164–177
  single vocal sources, 149–164
    for research, 149–155
  source of, 147–148
  studio, 150–151
    effects processing, 153–155
    problems, 153
  systems, 108–133
    microphone preamp stage, 108–113
Voiced sound source, 30, 39
Voiceless sound source, 30, 39

Voicing lead, defined, 49
Vowel quadrilateral, 36
Vowel sounds, **35**
Vowels
  identity loss of, **54**
  sound modifiers, 45–47

W

Wanted sound, **70**
  defined, 69
Waveforms, 8–10
  aperiodic, 10
  complex periodic, 10
Wavelength (λ), 7
Wide-band spectrogram, 16
Workstation, digital audio, 133

Y

Yottabytes (Yb), defined, 5

Z

Zettabytes (Zb), defined, 5
Zoomed acoustic waveforms, 9